Man Against Disease

OPUS General Editors

Keith Thomas *Humanities*
J. S. Weiner *Sciences*

J. A. Muir Gray

Man Against Disease

Preventive Medicine

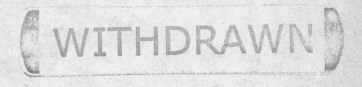

Oxford University Press 1979

Oxford New York Toronto Melbourne

Oxford University Press, Walton Street, Oxford OX2 6DP

OXFORD   LONDON   GLASGOW
NEW YORK   TORONTO   MELBOURNE   WELLINGTON
KUALA LUMPUR   SINGAPORE   JAKARTA   HONG KONG   TOKYO
DELHI   BOMBAY   CALCUTTA   MADRAS   KARACHI
NAIROBI   DAR ES SALAAM   CAPE TOWN

British Library Cataloguing in Publication Data

Gray, J A L Muir
    Man against disease.
    1. Medicine, Preventive
    I. Title
    614.4'4   RA425   78-41308

    ISBN 0-19-219140-3
    ISBN 0-19-289127-8 Pbk

*Printed in Great Britain by
Lowe and Brydone Printers Limited
Thetford, Norfolk*

Contents

To Jackie with love

Acknowledgements

It is impossible to name everyone who has contributed to this book. All who have taught me have influenced my thinking, as have those I have been fortunate enough to teach: the latter group have been more influential than they realize. Friends and colleagues in local and central government; in schools, colleges, and universities; in the National Health Service; in voluntary organizations, advertising, journalism, insurance, and commerce—all have helped me formulate my ideas. Of all this group I would like to mention especially Dr. Alex Gatherer, Dr. Peter Lawrence, and Dr. John Warin, who have supervised my work in public health, and Derek Lewis and Max Blythe who have taught me about health education.

I am most grateful to the following people, who generously gave their time to read and criticize the text: Lord Trend, Lord Briggs, Dr. S. Adam, Dr. J. Black, Mr. J. Guillebaud, Dr. W. Hamilton, Dr. P. Harker, Dr. L. Kinlen, Dr. D. Lane, Dr. J. Mann, Dr. A. Macfarlane, Dr. K. McPherson, Dr. M. Pelling, Dr. R. Peto, Dr. N. Wald, Dr. C. Webster, Ms. A. Hawker, Mr. P. Allen, Mr. S. Armson, Mr. W. Bradshaw, Mr. D. Charles-Edwards, Mr. M. Daube, and Mr. T. Fenn.

I would like to thank Sir George Pickering, who stimulated my interest in public health, Sir Richard Doll, whose writings have always inspired me, and Dr. Anthony Storr, who has encouraged me on many occasions. I am especially grateful for the help of my friend Howard Williams with whom many of the ideas discussed in this book have been hammered out. Extremely valuable comments were received from individuals working in the British Chest, Heart, and Stroke Association, The British Rheumatism and Arthritis Association, The Health and Safety Executive, Oxfam, The Royal Society for the Prevention of Accidents (RoSPA), and War On Want. Their comments, of course, do not imply that these organizations would necessarily endorse all the statements made in the text.

I wish to thank Mrs. J. Wilkins and Mr. S. Albert who translated my untidy manuscript into impeccable typescript, and my publishers who converted that typescript into this attractive text. There are so many people involved in the publication of a book whom the author never meets that it may appear invidious to single out two of those I did meet for special mention, but I cannot let the contributions of Adam Sisman and Judy Spours pass without recording my gratitude—they not only helped in the publication of the book but in its creation. I am also grateful for Andrew Schuller's continuing advice and encouragement.

I cannot express my gratitude to my wife adequately; she has helped in so many ways.

Any merits this book may be deemed to display are due to the influence of others. Any deficiencies are entirely my own.

The tables and graphs on pages 57, 77, 78, 79, 83, 87, 88, 100, 103, 124, 152, 156, 160 and 161 are reproduced with the permission of the Controller of Her Majesty's Stationery Office.

1 Prevention in the past

Anyone wishing to learn about the prevention of disease in times past will read in vain those history text books which are customarily used in schools, colleges, and universities. Not only prevention but the prevailing diseases receive little attention, with the exception of the Black Death. There are two principal reasons for this paucity of information.

Firstly, the sources of information about disease are often incomplete, and those which are complete are frequently inaccurate. Accurate, complete censuses are a comparatively recent innovation. The first census in Britain was not conducted until 1801, but by using all the available statistics it is possible to estimate the size of the population before this time, and the records suggest that it grew at an increasing rate, with some fluctuation in the rate of growth and a marked decrease in the population at the time of the plague, which may have even preceded the plague.

Although it is certain that the population increased, it is not possible to state with confidence how much of that growth was due to a decrease in the mortality rate and how much was due to an increase in the birth rate in the years before 1838. In that year, registration of births and deaths was introduced by the Civil Registration Act. It is only with this basic information that it is possible to estimate these determinants of population growth accurately, census information being insufficient. Thomas McKeown, Professor of Social Medicine at Birmingham University, has made estimates of the factors contributing to the population growth before 1838, but it is only after this year that they can be plotted with confidence.

The reasons for the fall in the birth rate after 1838 are still a matter of debate, as are the reasons for the decline in the death rate. It is generally accepted that the decline in mortality was principally due to a decrease in deaths from infectious diseases, but it remains uncertain which infectious diseases contributed most. McKeown

Population, birth rate, and death rate: England and Wales

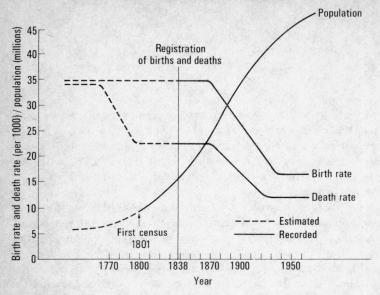

Source: McKeown & Lowe, *An Introduction to Social Medicine* (Blackwell, 1974) p. 6.

has proposed that a decline in tuberculosis deaths accounted for nearly one-half of the total decrease; typhus and typhoid for about a fifth; scarlet fever for a fifth; cholera, dysentery, and diarrhoea for nearly a tenth; and smallpox for one-twentieth. This remains, and will remain, a matter of conjecture, because the diagnosis of disease was often wrong in the nineteenth century. Diseases were confused with one another; for example, typhus was confused with typhoid, and some deaths were attributed to 'continued fever' which is not recognized today; and deaths listed under this rubric were probably due to other diseases such as typhoid. In earlier times errors of diagnosis and classification were even greater—it is recorded that in medieval times there was confusion between leprosy, syphilis, and smallpox. However, the paucity and inaccuracy of data is only one reason why most students of history are taught little about disease.

Another reason is that the majority of historians have been less interested in the affairs of everyday life, such as attitudes and beliefs, diet and diseases, than in political, ecclesiastical, and, more recently, economic history. Princes and popes, battles and treaties, have captured the imagination of successive generations of historians whereas the lives of common men and women have been unfashionable. It is true that there is often less accurate information about the lives and deaths of common people but much greater use could have been made of that which exists if historians had been more interested. This is changing. Increasing attention is being paid to social history, a trend which can also be determined in the history of medicine. The Wellcome Unit for the Study of the History of Medicine in Oxford and the Cambridge Group for the History of Population and Social Structure are two of the most prominent of a growing number of research units which have a particular interest in this aspect of the past. The research of such social historians allows a number of inferences to be drawn about the prevention of disease. These inferences must be treated with caution because of the deficiencies in the data on which they are based, but they suggest some principles of preventive medicine.

● **The decline in mortality can be attributed more to the prevention of disease than to the development of specific therapies.**

Before the nineteenth century there were very few effective therapies so it can be assumed that any decline in mortality must have been due to preventive measures. The improvement in mortality during the nineteenth century in Britain was due, in some part, to the growth of science and the introduction of some effective means of treatment. The principle of antisepsis and the practice of anaesthesia are two outstanding contributions to medicine, but in spite of the fact that the basic medical sciences, such as bacteriology and physiology, made great strides during the last century, their contribution to therapeutics was very small. In the twentieth century many effective cures have been developed, but most of this advance has taken place in the years following the Second World War during which no great improvement in the rate of increase in the expectation of life can be detected.

Expectation of life (in years) at birth in Britain, 1871–1971

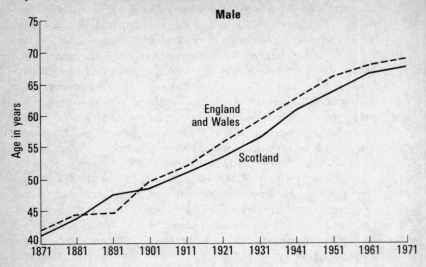

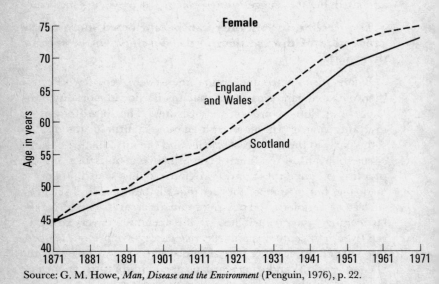

Source: G. M. Howe, *Man, Disease and the Environment* (Penguin, 1976), p. 22.

● Some diseases have declined spontaneously rather than as a result of man's actions.

Because a decrease in the mortality rate from a disease can always be associated with certain social changes which have taken place over the same period of time, it cannot be assumed that such social changes are the cause of the decrease in the death rate (see page 27). A decrease can occur due to a change in the relationship between man and the infecting micro-organism which causes the disease. Scarlet fever was a common cause of death in the nineteenth century and many adults in Britain can remember how serious it was before the Second World War. On the periphery of most cities were built fever hospitals which usually had one or more wards for scarlet fever cases. However, scarlet fever is now a mild disease which rarely causes death, although there have been few significant advances in its treatment. The decline in scarlet fever in both Britain and America is almost certainly a natural one, owing nothing to man's influence on the disease or the environment. The example of scarlet fever suggests that a natural decrease in the virulence of an infectious disease must always be considered when its mortality decreases. Such an evolutionary change in the genetic composition may have contributed to the decline in tuberculosis, plague, and leprosy.

Respiratory tuberculosis—mean annual death rate: England and Wales

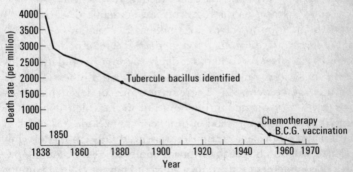

Source: T. McKeown and C. R. Lowe *An Introduction to Social Medicine* (Blackwell, 1974) p. 8.

If the time scale of the decline in mortality from tuberculosis is examined it is obvious that much of the decline was due to its prevention. It has been suggested that tuberculosis was prevented because there was an improvement in the nutritional status of the British people during this period, increasing their resistence to *Mycobacterium tuberculosis*, the micro-organism which causes the diseases, but other factors may also have been important. It is unlikely there was a significant change in the genetic composition of British people over such a short time, but it is possible that Mycobacterium tuberculosis itself changed, because bacteria reproduce much more frequently than humans.

Plague was unknown in Britain before 1348, when it entered from Europe at Weymouth in Dorset (see page 23). It cut through the population in four great swathes—the 'pestilences' of 1348–50, 1361–2, 1368–9, and 1375–6. The population of England was reduced from 3.8 to 2.5 million by the Black Death during this period and the effect in Europe was of similar magnitude; half of the 90,000 Florentines died. Epidemics recurred periodically until 1665, the year of the Great Plague, after which plague vanished from these islands and from Europe.

The term leprosy was probably applied to a large number of disfiguring illnesses but there is no doubt that the disease of leprosy caused by *Mycobacterium leprae*, a bacterium related to that which causes tuberculosis, was present in Britain continuously from the sixth century until the fifteenth century. It was what is termed an endemic disease, as distinct from an epidemic disease which affects a population in waves, like influenza. (Epidemic is derived from the Greek *epi*, meaning upon, and *demos*, meaning the people. An epidemic disease comes suddenly upon a population; an endemic disease is one which smoulders in it. Epidemiology is the study of epidemics). A great network of lazar houses—leprosaria—were opened throughout Europe in which lepers were confined. Over a long period of time leprosy became less and less common and all these lazar houses were gradually emptied during the fourteenth and fifteenth centuries, many of them becoming the houses of confinement for people who would now be called mentally ill, as Michel Foucault describes in *Madness and Civilisation*.

There may have been some change in European society which caused the disappearance of plague and leprosy, or their decline

may have been due to the introduction of conditions more favourable to other bacteria, such as Mycobacterium tuberculosis or
Treponema pallidum, the cause of syphilis, which displaced the
leprosy and plague bacteria from their previously stable position in
the ecosystem. Alternatively, there may have been genetic changes
in either the human hosts or in the infecting bacteria or, in the case
of plague, in one of the carriers of plague, the rat and the rat flea, so
that the balance of the biological relationship between man and
micro-organism shifted in favour of man. Bacteria reproduce so
quickly that genetic mutations occur not infrequently, but it is also
possible that the genetic composition of the human host changed
even in such a short period of time. Within any population there is
always a range of resistance to infection, some people being more
resistant than others. Leprosy was endemic for nine centuries and
as lepers were excluded from society and to an extent from marriage
and procreation many of the people who were more resistant to
leprosy may have selected one another in marriage. Such self-
selection breeding could have changed the genetic pool. Plague
prevailed in Britain for a much shorter period, for only three
centuries, but the mortality was so high that perhaps the more
susceptible members of society were culled and the more resistent
left to marry and pass on the genes which confer resistance. The
suggestion that the decline of the black rat *(Rattus rattus)* and its
replacement by the brown rat *(Rattus norvegicus)*, which lives less
close to man, was responsible for the decline is discounted by
W. H. McNeill in his stimulating book *Plagues and Peoples*. The
disappearance of these diseases remains a mystery. It is a possibility
that man was responsible for their decline either by his conscious
efforts, for example quarantine regulations to prevent the spread of
plague, or by his influence on some other aspect of life which
inadvertently led to their decline, but the possibility remains that
their decline was natural and cannot be attributed to man's
ingenuity and influence.

● **General improvements in the standard of living have had
as least as much to do with the decline in disease and mortality
as policies directed at the specific prevention of individual
diseases.**

The struggle for survival may be considered to be a form of

prevention, except that it is concerned with the prevention of premature death from deficiencies of the basic needs of life, shelter, warmth, water, and food, whereas the term preventive medicine concerns the prevention of premature death and disability from diseases. As society became progressively more skilled and better organized, so man came to be less affected by the vagaries of nature, its droughts, floods, and pests, and its members therefore less prone to die as a result of deficiencies of their primary needs. The transition from nomadic hunting to a settled pastoral life, the construction of granaries, the development of irrigation, the invention of the heavy, moldboard plough (the *carruca*), the introduction of three-crop rotation, the growth of trade and the increasing use of currency and credit have all improved the level of nutrition and buffered the effect of the normal fluctuations of climate and harvest yields. The balance of the food economy in the past was however always unstable. The climate was as fickle then as now and poor harvests were not uncommon, often followed by a second lean year because the supply of next year's seed corn was also affected by a bad harvest. People starved in lean years, but famine never caused large numbers of deaths directly; its influence was more frequently indirect. Malnutrition vitiates a population, rendering it susceptible to infection and making a fatal outcome of infection more probable.

The diet of Britain appears to have improved since 1601 but there have been times of hardship which, it is thought, were associated with epidemics of infectious disease. Typhus was a disease which was both endemic, that is it was continually present, and epidemic, although the history of this disease is uncertain as it was often confused with other diseases, especially the enteric fevers— typhoid and paratyphoid—which were so called because they cause similar symptoms (see page 3). The number of people affected by typhus increased very quickly in hard times because the resistance to infection was reduced by malnutrition. There had been epidemics in 1718, 1728, and 1741, each one following a bad harvest, and typhus was continuously endemic in the nineteenth century. The last and most severe epidemic occurred in 1846–8 and was, as always, associated with malnutrition. It was the aftermath of the Irish Potato Famine and was conveyed to Britain by Irishmen through Liverpool and Glasgow which was then, as now, the worst urban environment in Britain. An improvement in diet was probably also a contributory factor to the decline of tuberculosis in the nineteenth and twentieth centuries.

The nineteenth century was also a period during which the standard of housing improved, which may have contributed to the decline in typhus and tuberculosis, and during which the introduction of piped water and the disposal of sewage were responsible, at least in part, for the decrease in deaths due to typhoid, paratyphoid, cholera, diarrhoea, dysentery, and gastro-enteritis. These are all diseases caused by bacteria which spread by the contamination of water by human sewage.

Necessary though it is to emphasize the importance of general economic influences, the contribution of specific preventive measures should not be underestimated. Attempts to control the spread of infection by the isolation or hospitalization of infected people and those with whom they have had contact have played a part in the control of some diseases, for example smallpox, plague, and cholera. The word quarantine is derived from the Italian *quaranta* meaning forty, which is said to have been the duration of quarantine imposed on ships at Ragusa, and quarantine regulations were frequently imposed, though how effectively they were implemented is uncertain. Several Acts to prevent the spread of infectious diseases were passed in the nineteenth century; for example, the Nuisance Removal and Disease Prevention Act of 1846 increased the powers of 'any Town Councils or other like Body having Jurisdiction within any Corporate Town, Borough, City or Place' to effect 'the more speedy Removal of certain Nuisances, and to enable the Privy Council to make Regulations for the Prevention of contagious and epidemic Diseases'. In this century the World Health Organization has introduced systems of disease control aimed particularly at preventing the spread of yellow fever and smallpox by international travellers. This type of preventive measure is designed to prevent the spread of infection. The development of vaccination in the last two hundred years has taken prevention a step further—towards the prevention of infection itself.

The first disease prevented by vaccination was smallpox, a virus infection which spreads directly from man to man. The virus *Variola major* is inhaled and spreads throughout the body producing

its characteristic rash and toxaemia. It had been endemic in
Britain since the middle of the sixteenth century, smouldering
quietly until the eighteenth century during which there were
numerous epidemics. Edward Jenner was a Fellow of the Royal
Society, elected not for his work on smallpox but for his research on
the cuckoo, having been the first to propose that the hollow in the
back of the cuckoo fledgling was an adaptation for lifting the eggs
of the host bird over the edge of the nest. While engaged in his
biological research, Jenner noticed that cowmaids who had been
infected with cowpox, which was called Vaccinia, rarely contracted
smallpox. In 1796 he inoculated James Phipps, a Gloucestershire
boy, with fluid from a pox on the hand of Sarah Nelmes, a cowmaid.
The boy was protected and vaccination was introduced with
increasing enthusiasm. The Vaccination Act of 1840 empowered
the guardians or overseers of every parish or union in England and
Wales to pay doctors to perform free vaccination for those who
wished it. The second Vaccination Act of 1853 made the procedure
compulsory for infants within three months of birth and further
Vaccination Acts in 1871 and 1874 consolidated this legislation.
But the prevention of smallpox was not effected by legislation
alone; social change took place which led to greater public acceptance of vaccination and the compulsory powers of the Acts were
applied to only a minority of the public.

Over 100 years elapsed between Jenner's discovery that the
injection of cowpox material reduced the risk of infection by smallpox and the introduction of vaccination against other diseases. In
the interval it was discovered that the injection of a harmless strain
of bacteria, which had similar physical and chemical properties to
those of a species of bacteria which causes disease, stimulated the
body's immune system to make proteins called antibodies which
attack and destroy both the injected harmless bacteria and any
virulent bacteria of the related species which might subsequently
enter the body.

Vaccines routinely used in Britain

Tuberculosis	B.C.G.—Bacille Calmette Guérin—a live but weakened strain of tuberculosis bacteria.
Polio	Live weakened polio virus.

Diphtheria	Diphtheria toxoid (inactivated toxin); the harmful effects of diphtheria bacteria result from the chemical toxin they produce.
Pertussis (whooping cough)	Dead pertussis bacteria.
Measles	Live weakened measles virus.
Rubella (German measles)	Live weakened rubella virus.
Tetanus	Tetanus toxoid (inactivated toxin); the harmful effects of tetanus bacteria result from the toxin they produce.

Since the introduction of vaccination these diseases have certainly declined, but when set against a longer time scale their effect appears less important. In Professor McKeown's opinion— 'It seems probable that immunization has had a substantial effect on the reduction of deaths from smallpox and diphtheria, and more recently on the smaller problems of poliomyelitis and (less certainly) tetanus. The effective procedures were too late to have much influence on two of the most important causes of death— tuberculosis and whooping cough—and they have had no effect at all on the trend of mortality from measles.'

Diphtheria. Mean annual death rate of children under 15: England and Wales

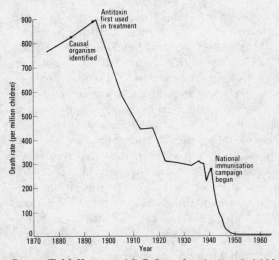

Source: T. McKeown and C. R. Lowe *Introduction to Social Medicine* (Blackwell, 1974) p. 92.

Whooping cough. Mean annual death rate of children under 15: England and Wales

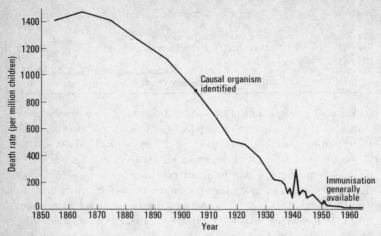

Source: T. McKeown and C. R. Lowe *Introduction to Social Medicine* (Blackwell, 1974) p 97.

Until recently, vaccination was generally accepted by parents. In some parts of the country almost every child was vaccinated, but publicity given to the adverse effects of whooping cough vaccine, and the manner in which the Department of Health appeared to have obfuscated the facts led to suspicion and a drop in the vaccination rate. In 1977 less than half the children at risk were immunized against whooping cough and in 1978 a minor epidemic developed, probably a consequence of the lower immunization rate which derived from a change in parental attitude towards vaccination. Just as attitudes towards smallpox vaccination were influenced in the nineteenth century by the realization that a safe preventive measure was available for a common dangerous disease so, in the 1970s, parents came to regard whooping cough vaccination as a potentially dangerous procedure designed to prevent what was, by then, a rare disease. Specific preventive measures are not only affected by the general physical environment of the times but by the prevailing climate of social opinion.

● **Poverty has always been a common preventable cause of disease.**

Statistical data are numerical generalizations. They summarize certain characteristics of groups of people, but in so doing they inevitably hide the characteristics of each individual and often mask the fact that there are distinct sub-groups within the main group. The figure calculated for the whole group in the type of statistics commonly used is on averages which do not indicate the range of values within the group. For example, the Infant Mortality Rate (the number of babies dying per 1,000 live births per year) calculated for Scotland in 1961 did not reveal the range of infant mortality in different social classes, from 17.4 in social classes I and II (professional and managerial) to 30.0 in social classes IV and V (partly skilled and unskilled). The decline in mortality discussed so far hides the differences in the rate of decline in different social and occupational classes in Britain, and in different age groups— the infant mortality rate did not start to decline until the end of the nineteenth century, some thirty years after the decline in overall mortality commenced. During the nineteenth century comparatively little attention was paid to such disparities but in its last decade, and in the first decade of the twentieth century, a number of studies demonstrated that the improvement in child health had not paralleled that in adult health, and that health problems were more common among poor people than among those who were materially more prosperous. In the early years of the new century Charles Booth's *Life and Labour of the People of London* was influential and Seebohm Rowntree reported his findings in York in *Poverty: A Study of Town Life,* both of which described the extent and effects of poverty. An Inter-Departmental Committee on Physical Deterioration, which had been set up by the government because one half of those young men who volunteered for Boer War Service had had to be rejected due to ill health and unsatisfactory physique, reported in 1904. Its findings were shocking, revealing that over one-third of children were malnourished and the new school health service recorded similar findings (see page 58). Of great importance in this re-awakening of public interest in disease and the need for prevention were Sidney and Beatrice Webb who edited, and largely wrote, a Minority Report on the evidence submitted to the Royal Commission on the Poor Laws and Relief of Distress which sat from 1905 to 1909. They proposed radical changes to tackle the problems of poverty and inequality and to improve the health of children and poor people by personal preventive medicine. The State had first significantly acknowledged personal poverty in 1601 with the passing of the Elizabethan Poor Law. This Act, and the Amending Acts which followed in the course of the next three centuries, were drafted to deal with the financial problems, paying little attention to the cause, or causes, which had impoverished the individual. Old people, those who were disabled or suffered from mental illness, unemployed people, and deserted mothers, were all treated in the same way by the 1601 Poor Law; subjected to a means test and offered either outdoor or indoor relief in the workhouse. In the nineteenth century steps were taken to recognize the distinct problems of people who were physically or mentally ill, but the basic principles of the now outmoded Poor Law were not seriously questioned until the Webbs' Minority Report challenged the conclusions of the Majority Reports which, in the Webbs' opinion, left the underlying causes of poverty untouched and perpetuated the Poor Law principles. It could be argued that the Webb's analyses were too gloomy. A succession of Acts placed on the Statute Book in the years between the turn of the century and the final repeal of the Poor Law by the National Assistance Act of 1948 were designed to tackle the causes of poverty not only by means of financial support, such as old age pensions, but by the provision of services, such as school meals and the school health service. However, there are still disadvantaged people in every society and their health problems are, in general, greater than those who have a larger share of the State's wealth (see page 152). Wealth alone does not ensure health. Although some diseases become less common if people become wealthier, others increase. It is not wealth alone which prevents disease but the use which is made of it. This depends on many factors, but it seems justifiable to infer from the evidence of the past that the prevention of disease cannot be considered in isolation from the economic and political nature of society, and that social and political inequalities have to be tackled as well as the introduction of specific preventive measures, if prevention is to reach its full potential.

● **No single factor was responsible for the upsurge of interest in disease prevention during the first half of the nineteenth century or for the continuing growth of interest since then.**

Within this diffuse pattern of social change there are occasions when the sequence of change can be identified as a discrete process, particularly when individuals have been damaged or have died in a fashion which allows them to be portrayed almost as martyrs. For example, the damage caused by thalidomide was a very important stimulant to the changes leading to better, albeit by no means ideal, scrutiny of the safety of new drugs (see page 49). Similarly the small number of deaths of people working with asbestos have led to a series of government initiatives to protect workers and consumers from this particular substance. Nevertheless, these are exceptions. In general, the various preventive measures which have been introduced have to be viewed as part of a coherent social process rather than as a collection of unrelated responses to individual problems.

The prevention of disease became a prominent social issue in the first half of the nineteenth century but the origins of this shift in public policy can be traced much further back. The change took place partly because people were stimulated by new knowledge and new epidemics; public attitudes were shaped by the prevailing diseases. Tuberculosis was the commonest cause of death when Victoria came to the throne and the first report of the Registrar General attributed 17.6 per cent of all deaths to tuberculosis. Associated with poor diet and bad housing, tuberculosis, known as consumption or phthisis, was greatly feared, yet perhaps because it was ubiquitous and perennial it evoked much less reaction than typhus and cholera which occurred in epidemics.

Typhus was both endemic and epidemic. It had been continuously present for hundreds of years, but the number of people affected by typhus increased very quickly in hard times because the resistance to infection was reduced by malnutrition (see page 8). Terrible though typhus was, it did not seem to create as much public concern as did cholera which occurred in Britain for the first time in the nineteenth century.

Cholera spreads from one individual to another either directly or by contamination of water, the bacterium *Vibrio cholerae* causing severe diarrhoea and death from dehydration. Cholera spread from its Asian source through Afghanistan, Persia, and Europe along trade routes. In 1831 William IV opened Parliament with a grave announcement of the 'continued progress of a

formidable disease'. Four months later in October 1831 it reached
Hamburg, and the first case in Britain was diagnosed in the port of
Sunderland on 4 November. Four great epidemics followed in
1832, 1848–9, 1853–4, and 1866, throwing the whole country into
turmoil. In *Cholera 1832*, R. J. Morris suggests that the terror and
the lessons of the first attack were soon forgotten, but cholera could
not be forgotten for long and the recurrent epidemics contributed
to a change in public opinion and the need for a better environment.
The relative importance of typhus and cholera as agents of social
change is uncertain. Although typhus was more frequently men-
tioned in the debates leading to the 1848 Public Health Act the
evidence, presented by Norman Longmate in *King Cholera*, of the
terror and riots which followed cholera makes it probable that it
was equally important. Because cholera was new and alien it
evoked a range of emotional responses from the public which
influenced their attitudes. Not all responses were conducive to
prevention. There was opposition to some of the measures proposed
and taken but the conflict between certain sections of the public
and the authorities created a tension which probably furthered the
prevention debate, and led to the acceptance of the need for
preventive legislation. Social change does not take place in
indifference.

The contribution of new knowledge is more difficult to assess. In
spite of the fact that the nineteenth century saw the birth of
bacteriology, pathology, and physiology, new knowledge appears
to have contributed comparatively little to the pressure for change.
Pasteur's theory of germs was not soundly established until a
decade after the first Public Health Act. John Snow did indeed
remove the handle from the water pump in Soho's Broad Street,
demonstrating the link between water and cholera by the fact that
no more cases of cholera developed in the surrounding area which
had hitherto been heavily infected, but this was in 1853 and his
theory took many more years to be universally accepted over the
popular theory that cholera was carried by a miasma of foul air.
Legislators operated on the principle enunciated by Sir John Simon
that 'the interests of health and the interests of common physical
comfort and convenience are in various cases identical'. Anything
which affected comfort and convenience—an accumulation of
sewage, verminous dwellings, or the keeping of pigs near human

habitation—was deemed to be a nuisance and a risk to health. The title of the 'Nuisance Removal and Disease Prevention' Acts epitomizes this principle which was sound but not based on scientific evidence.

It is, however, oversimplified to imagine that science and social change were not related to one another. The influence of science should not be underestimated although there are few examples of newly discovered scientific facts leading directly to social change. The eighteenth century enlightenment had changed man's view of the world and his position in it. There were still those who saw cholera as divine retribution for the depravity of the times, but the idea that the body was a physico-chemical system and that illnesses had physico-chemical causes was widely accepted. Religion remained an important influence, but nineteenth-century man was more able to appreciate arguments about causality. This was not a new ability. Anthropologists have revealed how societies of simple technology can simultaneously handle concepts of scientific causality and religious predestination, for example in B. Malinowski's *Science, Magic and Religion*. There is also evidence that, although society's interpretation of the plague was strongly influenced by their views of theodicy, people took many preventive measures because they accepted that an individual's infection came from another individual. In the nineteenth century, however, the influence of science became much stronger than the influence of a religious theodicy.

Stimulants for change are not enough. Society must be in a state of preparedness, ready to be stimulated. In part the readiness of society in the nineteenth century to accept the ideas of prevention can be explained by their different views of the physical world, as described above, but there were other social and philosophical changes which prepared the way for change. The steadily growing involvement of the State in disease prevention over the last one-hundred-and-fifty years has been in parallel with its increasing influence in other aspects of life. This trend is not only a consequence of secularization, the decline in ecclesiastical power from the beginning of the nineteenth century to the present day. There has been a real growth in State intervention. This can be interpreted as being the result of the prevailing political philosophies of this era, during which concepts of distributive justice have changed and equality has become a politically important issue. The slow growth in power of classes previously impotent, invoked by the spread of the franchise, and the rise of trade unionism has influenced styles of government. Not all people who could be called working class welcomed public health and other welfare legislation. Occasionally some reacted violently to moves which they construed as having been designed to make them healthier only to allow them to be worked harder. Conversely, not everyone of those who had wealth and power to lose resisted these social changes. The revolutionary spirit in the late eighteenth and early nineteenth centuries provided a climate of opinion in which health became an important issue and the political trends since then have been such as to increase its importance.

There has been a shift in the attitudes and values which has influenced all classes, but change cannot come from good intentions alone. It requires wealth sufficient to pay for the necessary changes and a bureaucracy stable and honest enough to implement them. The rise of interest in prevention took place at a time of economic and technological advance without which progress would have been much more difficult.

Essential for change to occur are *changeurs*, those individuals and groups who have the commitment and ability to release the potential energy for change. The public health movement had a number of outstanding campaigners, such as Lord Shaftesbury, John Simon, Florence Nightingale, Thomas Southwood Smith, and Edwin Chadwick. Committed, opinionated, and abrasive, Chadwick was very influential but he made powerful enemies, including *The Times*. As Secretary of the Poor Law Commission he was the main author of the Report on the Sanitary Conditions of the Labouring Population of Great Britain, published in 1842, and was appointed to the General Board of Health in 1848, but his abrasive manner impaired its effectiveness and when the Board was reconstituted in 1854 he lost his seat.

The laws were implemented at local level due to the activities of Medical Officers of Health and Inspectors of Nuisances, who became Sanitary Inspectors in 1921, Public Health Inspectors in 1956, and Environmental Health Officers in 1974. In the same year as part of the reorganization of the National Health Service, the title of Medical Officer of Health was replaced by the District

Community Physician or Specialist in Community Medicine for Environmental Health who is no longer employed by the local authority but by the health service—a subtle but significant change.

All these factors interrelate; the growth of interest in prevention is a reflection of a number of different social themes. If one can be said to have been the unifying theme it was the growing respect for the rights and welfare of the individual although, paradoxically, steps to establish this principle in practice have led to a growth in the power of the State at the expense of the individual.

● **The growing power of the state and the medical profession has facilitated the prevention of disease and, in the process of prevention, the power of the State and the medical profession has been further increased. Similarly the centralization of power has facilitated the prevention of disease and moves to prevent disease have contributed to the centralization of power.**

Although individual states had taken steps to prevent disease before the nineteenth century, for example by the imposition of quarantine on ships, it was during that century that prevention by the use of public authority grew significantly, being marked by a series of Parliamentary Acts. The Public Health Act of 1848 instituted the first General Board of Health and made statutory the setting up of local Boards of Health in districts in which the death rate was greater than twenty-three per thousand inhabitants. The Nuisance Removal and Disease Prevention Act of 1848 dealt with the immediate problems of the second cholera epidemic. In 1852 the Metropolis Water Act proscribed the extraction of water from the Thames below Teddington. The Sanitary Act of 1866 was a response to the fourth cholera epidemic. Another Public Health Act in 1871 created the system of surveillance at ports to prevent the importation of disease, and a consolidating Act was placed on the Statute Book in 1875 by Disraeli's Government which divided the country into urban and rural sanitary districts, each of which was obliged to appoint a Medical Officer of Health. Many other Acts were introduced, for example the Housing of the Working Classes Act of 1885, the Local Government Act of 1888, and the Infectious Diseases Act of 1889—which were intended to prevent disease resulting from an insanitary or polluted environment and noxious working conditions.

Although there was considerable legislative activity its effects are difficult to assess—Acts of Parliament are not initiators of social change. They are often modelled on procedures already in operation in one or more local areas and they usually reflect opinions held by importent sections of the community. Legislation often follows and consolidates change rather than causing it. This welter of new laws also reflected the growth of central authority in many other spheres which took place during the nineteenth century. Opposition to these laws was sometimes based on self-interest, for example, the resistance of those who owned the water companies to laws which seemed to be leading to the public ownership of waterworks, but another strong reason was a suspicion of centralization.

In the twentieth century the State's involvement in prevention has continued to expand, the provision of water and the disposal of sewage had become part of the infrastructure of society and has been increasingly taken for granted, but new hazards have required new measures. In this century the state has also tried to prevent poverty and its consequences, and it has provided a range of preventive health and social services for the individual. A whole series of Acts were passed to improve child and mother care. The Midwives Act of 1902 improved the standard of midwifery, The Education (Provision of Meals) Act of 1906 improved nutrition, the 1907 Education Act saw the start of the school medical service which offered free inspection and treatment to children. In 1915 the Notification of Births Act made compulsory the notification of every birth to the Medical Officer of Health. Notification mobilized the health visiting service, which had grown from several beginnings in Birmingham, Liverpool, Manchester, and Salford to a well organized local authority service ensuring that health visitors paid early visits to the newborn. In 1918 the Maternity and Child Welfare Act and the Education Act consolidated many of the previous steps and provided the basis of a service which has continued, largely unaltered, until the present day.

Personal preventive medicine was not only offered to mothers and children; in 1912 the local authority tuberculosis service was started, and in 1917 a similar service was set up for the prevention and treatment of venereal disease. The underlying problem of poverty and unsatisfactory housing was tackled by a whole variety of measures of which the most important were the introduction of National Health Insurance in 1911 and the series of Housing Acts which received Royal Assent in the early 1920s. This trend towards the provision of services for individuals was consolidated by the introduction of comprehensive financial benefits, by the National Assistance Act, and the National Health Service in 1948. There have been many innovations since then, such as the development of family planning services and the new approach to abortion, but the major steps in the provision of personal preventive services had been taken in the midst and aftermath of the Second World War.

Strong centralized public authorities have enabled these initiatives to be implemented and both central government and local authorities have grown in size and power; in 1841 government expenditure was only 11 per cent of the Gross National Product; by 1977 it was nearly one half. There has also been a tremendous growth of public expenditure in real terms. In 1900 it was £2.3 billion (1970 prices); by 1980 it is estimated that it will be more than £25 billion.

Not only did a stronger more centralized system of authority contribute to the prevention of disease but the converse holds true. The moves to prevent disease and premature death accelerated the process of centralization and strengthened the hand of public authority. Health became of political importance not only for its intrinsic appeal but as a symbol. A new approach was taken to distributive justice in the late eighteenth and nineteenth centuries. Egalitarianism grew to be a major political idea, at times discussed in terms of equality and justice, at other times in terms of health and disease, which became symbols of justice and injustice. The public health movement of the nineteenth century has to be viewed in the context of the other political and philosophical currents of that time. The same holds true in the twentieth century. The National Health Service was not only a means of treating disease, it was also a means of expressing certain fundamental ideals of the Labour movement. The inception of the National Health Service is a paradigm of the manner in which health matters increase the centralist tendency. To prevent unnecessary disability and premature death the idea of a National Health Service was conceived. For the idea of the NHS to be realized required not only a strong central government, but an increase in the size and strength of the centre. Also, when it was evident, even to the medical profession, that the NHS was a success it became another piece of evidence in favour of centralization. In the same way, the accurate and complete collection of mortality and sickness data only became possible when the central government reached a certain level of control, but the regional disparities revealed by such data, not only with respect to mortality (see page 153) but to other measures such as the unemployment levels, argued for more central control to distribute resources to regions in most need to satisfy egalitarian principles.

The same relationship can be detected between the medical profession and prevention. As medicine laid more secure empirical foundations on the findings of scientific research, and as it had an increasing number of effective therapies to offer, it became more authoritative. Although the medical profession was not always unanimous in its views on prevention it became increasingly influential. Certain doctors were delegated special powers as Medical Officers of Health; from 1848 any town could employ a Medical Officer of Health but the appointment was only made obligatory by the Public Health Act of 1872.

Not only did the medical profession increasingly influence and implement preventive measures but the burgeoning interest in health and the prevention of disease helped to augment the power and influence of the medical profession.

● **Man's modification of his environment has prevented many diseases but it has often created the conditions in which these diseases flourished: man brings diseases upon himself.**

Although self-inflicted diseases such as those caused by cigarette smoking or by the excessive consumption of alcohol or calories are sometimes considered as modern phenomena, many diseases which were formerly common were also caused by man's behaviour. The building of settled colonies and permanent houses, irrigation, domestication of animals, urbanization, the growth of trade, and industrialization are some of the trends which have played a central part in man's growth and development, but which have also brought disease. Plague, for example, came to Europe as a consequence of man's activities. Plague, the Black Death, is caused by infection by the bacterium *Pasteurella pestis,* either in the lungs as pneumonic plague or in the lymph nodes as bubonic plague. The bacteria are conveyed from man to man by the rat, the rat flea, and the human flea, such intermediary carriers of infection being called vectors. Plague was unknown in Europe until the Mongol's westward thrust for conquest carried their influence into Asia Minor. In 1346 the Tartars laid seige to Genoese merchants in Caffa, now called Feodesia, whither they had gone in their eastward quest for trade. As the Mongol troops died of plague, which had spread west along the trade routes, their bodies were catapulted into the city. The disease gained a foothold and was carried on the galleys to Genoa, thence to northern Europe.

Although its effects were not so devastating as those of plague, typhus was a new phenomenon in Europe in the eigthteenth century as plague had been in the fourteenth. The micro-organism which causes typhus, *Rickettsia prowazeki*, is transferred from man to man by a vector, the human louse, *Pediculus humanus humanus*. As it is associated with louse infestation typhus was, and is, a disease which flourishes where poverty, malnutrition, and overcrowding prevail, as they did in the growing cities of eighteenth-century Britain. The cities provided ideal conditions, not only for the spread of typhus, but for tuberculosis, smallpox, typhoid, para-typhoid, measles, diphtheria, scarlet fever, and gastro-enteritis.

Whenever man upsets the balance of the ecosystem in which he lives he may inadvertently create conditions in which new diseases may increase. Much publicity is now given to iatrogenic disease—that which is caused by doctors. Much more significant, in both past and present, is homogenic disease—that which is caused by man.

2   The scope for prevention today

Tools of prevention

Facts are the tools of preventive medicine—facts about causation. While curative medicine tackles the effects of diseases, preventive medicine is concerned with causes, and the causes of a disease are collectively called its aetiology. The simplest aetiology is infection by an agent which spreads directly from human to human, for example measles. The measles virus spreads easily, being carried in droplets of liquid in exhaled air. If the virus-laden droplet is inhaled by another person who has not previously been infected, the virus multiplies and spreads within the body. The effect of infection depends upon the number of viruses inhaled and the state of health of the individual who plays host to the infecting agent. A healthy child in Britain infected with measles may not even show a rash; a malnourished child in central Africa may die. The effect of infection is also influenced by the genetic composition of the individual infected. In populations in which measles has been endemic for centuries, as in Britain, the genetic pool has adapted to the effects of measles infection and it is a mild disease. In populations in which measles have never been known, the effects of introduction can be dramatic and serious. When measles was accidently introduced into Fiji in 1875 over 20,000 people—one quarter of the population—died. As the genetic composition of a population or an individual cannot be altered over a short period of time prevention can only be achieved by breaking the chain of infection by immunizing individuals or by improving the state of nutrition of people who are at risk of infection. With man to man infection the chain can be simply broken, provided that the infecting agent can be isolated so that a vaccine can be made, or there is sufficient wealth or political commitment to improve the state of nutrition of those at risk.

When the chain of infection from man to man involves other

species as vectors, prevention becomes more difficult, especially if the infecting agent has a life cycle with several stages. Although one factor can still be identified as 'the cause', the infecting agent, a number of other factors contribute to the aetiology. Such is the aetiology of schistosomiasis, which is also called bilharziasis (or Bill Harris as it was known by the Eighth Army). Man becomes infected by the larval forms (cercariae) of one of a number of species of the genus of trematode worm *Schistosoma* if they penetrate his skin while he is bathing or swimming in infected water. The male and female worms breed in the infected person's veins and the eggs are excreted in both urine and faeces to hatch in the water of lakes and streams, releasing the first larval form (miracidia) which enter certain species of snails, the vectors. The miracidia become cercariae, which leave the snail after several weeks able to infect man once more. The chain of causation can be broken and the disease prevented in a number of ways:

- The disposal of faeces and urine so that they will not contaminate water.
- Improved land drainage to reduce the breeding grounds of the snail.
- The use of chemicals to kill the snails.
- The provision of protective footwear and clothing for those exposed to contaminated water.
- The provision of a separate uncontaminated water supply for drinking and washing.
- Education of people at risk.
- Treatment of all infected people.

To adopt all these measures would be both time-consuming and expensive, and the technique of mathematical modelling has been introduced to help decide which factor should be tackled. At each stage in the life cycle of the trematode worm there are a number of variable factors. Some are controllable, for example the area of water in which snails can breed; others, such as the genetic constitution of the population at risk, are not. Each of these variables can be expressed mathematically, allowing the whole life cycle to be expressed as a formula, and the effects of employing the various preventive measures, alone or in combination, can be calculated. The technique is complicated, requiring the use of differential equations, but it has been facilitated by the use of computers.

The solutions to such equations are not predictions because every factor cannot be determined exactly—they are statements of probability. The life cycle of the trematode is not like the cycle of a planet's orbit; it cannot be precisely determined and the mathematical model cannot therefore be considered to be a deterministic model. Similarly the rate of worm reproduction cannot be precisely predicted if the number of worms in the body is low. An average reproduction rate of *schistosoma* worms can be calculated, but the reproduction rate of different worms rarely equals the average. The distribution of these values about the average is random, but a value can be calculated for the reproductive rate making allowance for the randomness of the distribution of the reproduction rates above and below the average rate. The mathematical model is not deterministic, it is what mathematicians call a stochastic model. Such a model allows those who are trying to prevent a disease to estimate what might be the most efficient and effective way of spending their available resources with greater accuracy than by making decisions intuitively. So far the emphasis has been on environmental modification—the introduction of better sanitation and water supplies—but this approach to prevention is only in its infancy. This emphasizes once more that diseases can be prevented by influencing a factor other than the infecting agent or the human host, and this may happen inadvertently. The intensive agriculture of the countryside around Rome between the sixth and third centuries B.C. involved the draining of swamps which prevented malaria from reaching the city, contributing among other factors to the rise of the Roman Empire.

Infectious disease can be considered to have a unifactoral aetiology. Although a number of factors are involved, only one factor, the infecting agent, initiates the disease process. In its absence disease will not occur. Measles cannot develop unless the virus is inhaled, nor can schistosomiasis unless a trematode worm of the appropriate species invades the body. The aetiology of non-infectious diseases is different because there is almost always more than one factor operating simultaneously in the initiation of the disease process. It sometimes appears that non-infectious disease is unifactoral, for example when someone whose blood alcohol level is much higher than the legal limit of 80 mgm per cent is injured because his car leaves the road. Although the amount of alcohol drunk is an important factor in such a road traffic accident and may have been the critical factor, there are always others such as the condition of the road surface, the quality of street lighting, the thickness of the tyre treads, and the driver's familiarity with the road, all of which are operating simultaneously. Non-smokers also develop lung cancer, so there must be other causes, such as the inhalation of radioactive dust, and some heavy smokers do not develop lung cancer so the relationship between lung cancer and smoking is not unifactoral as is the relationship between the invasion of the trematode worm and the development of schistosomiasis. The aetiology of non-infectious disease is said to be multi-factoral which makes the elucidation of its aetiology more difficult.

The search for causes of heart disease, the commonest killer in Britain and other developed countries, demonstrates this problem and the approaches which can be used to overcome it. The death rate from heart disease has increased steadily this century and it seems certain that this is a true increase. There has been neither an increase in the accuracy with which the diagnosis is made or recorded on the death certificate, nor any change in the way in which the term heart disease is understood and used by doctors, which could explain this escalation in the death rate as being due to other than an absolute increase in the number of men dying of heart disease. The increase has been so rapid, and heart disease now affects so many people, that it is often called an epidemic, although it is not an infectious disease. To explain this increase the epidemiologist has to consider the other changes which have taken place during this period. They are innumerable. Compared with 1948, for example, more people drive motor cars, more aeroplanes pollute the atmosphere, the amount of sugar, meat, and fat in the diet has increased, more books and scientific journals are published, more cigarettes are smoked, more people watch television, more wine is drunk, and there have been a host of other changes. The first step taken by the epidemiologist is to calculate which of the other changes, increases or decreases, bear a statistically significant relationship to the increase in heart disease. For each relationship a correlation coefficient can be calculated which expresses mathematically the relationship between the rate of increase in heart attack and the rate of change of each of these factors. Many of the relationships are statistically significant, that is to say it is improbable that the close correlation between the two rates of change has occurred by chance. Not all statistically significant relationships of them are causal, that is, responsible for the increase. Most of them are coincidental and have no connection with heart disease, and common sense and intelligence suggest that many are so. It is improbable that the increase in the rate of publishing the printed word has been a cause. It is also improbable that either motor cars or television cause heart disease directly, but both are associated with a decrease in the amount of exercise taken, and as exercise affects the heart its lack can be placed on the list of possible risk factors for further investigation.

The second step is to consider each possible risk factor on its own. For example, having established that there is a significant correlation coefficient between the increase in the consumption of cigarette tobacco and the increase in heart disease, the nature of the relationship, whether is it causal or coincidental, can be explored by comparing the rate of disease in people who smoke cigarettes with the rate in people who are identical in age, sex, race, occupation, and every other aspect which it is possible to identify and feasible to match, excepting that they do not smoke cigarettes. Having identified these two groups it may be possible to decide immediately whether the difference is such that cigarette smoking is a cause of heart disease or not. Alternatively the two groups may have to be observed for years to collect sufficient information.

In practice it is often very difficult to draw two such samples from the population being studied. Not only do humans vary from one another in very many aspects, but the distribution of other risk factors than the one under scrutiny can confuse the results. Although it is possible to divide a population into smokers and non-smokers, other possible risk factors such as the consumption of large amount of fat, high blood pressure, obesity, or physical inactivity may predominate in either the group of smokers or in the non-smokers, or be shared equally between the two groups. Any excess of heart disease which can be demonstrated in the group who smoke cannot be attributed to smoking unless these other factors are taken into account, which can be done by a mathematical technique called multivariate analysis, which allows each risk factor to be considered independently.

It should be emphasized that even if the relationship of a factor to the probability of illness is *not* statistically significant, that does not mean that it is *not* a cause of the disease. Although the Royal College of Physicians and the British Cardiac Society could neither find 'reliable evidence' that obesity was a risk factor nor 'definite evidence' that physical exercise prevented heart disease, they recommend that obesity be reduced and exercise increased on the evidence of their experience and clinical judgement. Such advance, based on intuition, not on statistically tested evidence, may be proved wrong, but it is frequently used because the empirical foundations of preventive medicine are still weak (see page 151).

Those searching for causes, the epidemiologists, process the information collected by government departments and other agencies. Ideas developed from such information may be tested in more detail by the results of surveys designed by the epidemiologist to answer one specific question. For example, Sir Richard Doll and Austin Bradford Hill conducted a postal questionnaire survey of the smoking habits of doctors and compared them with the causes of death registered when the doctors in the survey eventually died.

If facts are the tools of prevention, epidemiologists are the toolmakers. Epidemiologists are usually doctors of medicine who have specialized in the necessary intellectual approach and the mathematical skills which are required. Sir Richard Doll and the team working in Oxford, Bradford Hill in London, Archie Cochrane in Cardiff, and Jerry Morris in London, can be regarded as the pioneers of this new medical speciality. Epidemiologists work for the National Health Service, in universities and in special units, such as those run by the M.R.C., the Medical Research Council, and the London School of Hygiene and Tropical Medicine, which has contributed so much to the medical problems of under-developed countries. Mathematics cannot solve all the problems of preventive medicine, it cannot illuminate what Proust called 'the reasons of sentiment or the avoidable imprudences which may have led some particular person to his death', and epidemiologists now work with sociologists and anthropologists to uncover the reasons why people smoke cigarettes, overeat, and continue with behaviour that they know increases their probability of illness. The tools needed for the future are not only facts about causation but an understanding of the motives which influence human behaviour.

The need for prevention

During the 1960s man's enthusiasm for medicine was uninhibited and uncritical, as was his enthusiasm for science as a whole. The 1970s have, however, seen the development of a new, critical mood. Doubts have been expressed about the effectiveness of modern curative medicine, to what degree it actually achieves its stated ends, its efficiency, and at what cost those treatments which are effective are achieved. Cost, in this case, is assessed not only in pounds and pence but in terms of what else could be done with the resources used. For example, heart transplantation, the phenomenon of 1967 and 1968, was greeted with enthusiasum because it was a great technical achievement, but calmer consideration revealed that it was of only limited effectiveness, that it did not keep people alive for long periods of time, and that it was an inefficient procedure as it used large amounts of resources which could have been spent to greater effect on other treatments. Medicine was also criticized on the grounds that it had come to intrude too much in lives of individuals and had become too influential in society. Ivan Illich is the most eloquent proponent of this argument, and in *Medical Nemesis: The Expropriation of Health* he delivered a swingeing attack on medicine, opening his case with the uncompromising statement that 'the medical establishment has become a major threat to health. The disabling impact of professional control over medicine has reached the proportions of an epidemic.'

Medicine is not only under external attack; doctors themselves are now more sceptical and self-critical than formerly. Not only are they questioning the effectiveness of what they do—whether or not their treatments have any beneficial effects—but they are also concerned about the side-effects of and psychological dependence upon drugs and doctors that patients often develop—whether treatment is actually harmful. In this era of criticism and self-criticism, it is important not to under-estimate the contribution medicine has made in the last thirty years. The expectation of life has increased and many treatments have contributed to an improved quality of life, the cardiac pacemaker and the artificial hip being striking examples of effective high technology medicine. It is because it has become so effective in the prevention of pain, disability, and premature death that medicine has become prominent in society.

As it grows more effective it becomes less efficient; increasing investment in health services brings diminishing returns. With increasing investment comes an increasing incidence of iatrogenic disease, that which is caused by the action of doctors, such as the side-effects of drugs and the complications of surgical operations. Diseased tissue and healthy tissue are not in separate body compartments, they intermingle. The process of disease has many similarities to normal functioning, cancer cells have some of the characteristics of normal cells, and bacteria consist of similar chemicals to human cells, so the effects of treatment are not always specifically on the diseased tissue alone. As treatment affects diseased tissue more drastically, that is as it becomes more effective, its effects on normal tissue are sometimes also more drastic. Progress exacts its price. Nineteenth-century man may not have had antibiotics but neither did he have thalidomide, and this relationship between the effect of increasing investment in health services on the level of disease and its unwanted side-effects can be shown diagrammatically.

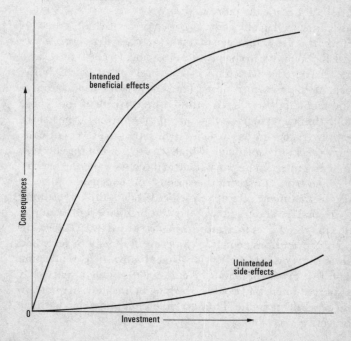

The position of developed countries can be plotted on the right-hand side. On a sound infrastructure with piped water, sewage disposal, good housing, and education, they are making increasingly heavy investment in health services with diminishing returns and an increasing incidence of iatrogenic disease. The position of under-developed countries (many cannot be said to be developing) is on the left side of the diagram. With low levels of investment in housing, water, sewage disposal, education or health services. They have high levels of disease but with little iatrogenic disease. Developed countries now have to consider preventive medicine not only because of the economic constraints on the expansion of curative services, but because many of these fatal and disabling conditions which are difficult, or impossible to cure are to some extent preventable. Although the major fatal and disabling conditions in developing countries, infectious diseases, are more frequently curable they too must consider prevention as these diseases so reduce the strength of the population that they cannot work, produce, and create the wealth necessary to strengthen the infrastructure and provide the more expensive health services. Now, as previously, the need in all countries is for a preventive approach.

It is important to emphasize that it is to some extent arbitrary to distinguish preventive from curative medicine, for the latter is also preventive. An effective clinician can prevent pain, disability, handicap, and premature death, and one view is that curative medicine should be considered within preventive medicine. Those who hold this view suggest that preventive medicine has three phases: primary preventive medicine, which tries to prevent disease; secondary preventive medicine, which tries to prevent the effects of disease by treatment at an early stage in its course; and the tertiary phase, which tries to prevent the serious consequences of disease by effective treatment. Curative medicine offers the opportunity for both secondary and tertiary preventive medicine. For example, the G.P. who recognizes that a sore throat is caused by streptococcal bacteria and prescribes penicillin can prevent rheumatic fever and rheumatic heart disease which sometimes follow such an infection (see page 74). Prevention and the curative medicine practised by general practitioners and doctors working in hospitals are not two different types of medicine. They are different approaches with the same objective.

This is demonstrated by the fall in the maternal mortality rate. Around the time at which the Royal College of Obstetricians and Gynaecologists was founded, in 1929, maternal mortality varied from forty to forty-five deaths for every 10,000 live births from one year to another. By 1975 the mortality rate had fallen to one death for every 10,000 live births. At first sight this appears to have been due to the introduction of blood transfusions and antibiotics, the improved treatment of pre-eclampsia (see page 53), and the tremendous improvement in the standard of obstetrics. However, the advance has been achieved not only by improved techniques but by the development of a preventive approach. Careful, regular ante-natal examinations offer properly trained doctors the opportunity to select high-risk cases for special care before problems arise—primary prevention, and the chance to detect problems at an early stage—secondary prevention. Hospital obstetrics is a form of preventive medicine, based on the same principles as general practice, health visiting and community midwifery, although it sometimes employs 'high technology' to achieve its objectives (see page 47).

The treatment of people with haemophilia also illustrates the artificiality of distinguishing preventive from curative medicine. Haemophilia is treated using the expensive products developed by the most advanced research methods by a small number of highly trained personnel workers in specialist units—high technology medicine. Yet this treatment is primarily preventive. It prevents death; disability and handicap; educational problems, by minimizing school absences; unemployment; and family breakdown.

It is as misleading to separate curative from preventive medicine as it is to imagine that hospital and community care are distinct services treating different types of problem. A hospital is a part of the community it serves. Effective curative medicine prevents pain, disability, and premature death and forms part of the spectrum of preventive medicine.

3 Opportunities in underdeveloped and developing countries

The wealth of nations and their health are interwoven like warp and woof. Nations which become wealthy can improve the public health by improving nutrition and by the provision of pure water, sewage disposal, housing, education, and health services to treat those citizens who fall ill.

However, nations which are affected by both endemic and epidemic diseases are in turn handicapped in the creation of wealth. Nations which have become successful and flourishing have been those in which disease was relatively less common than in those which failed to grow. The main factors favouring certain groups in early times were the climate and environment in which they lived. In the millennia before the birth of Christ the great civilizations developed in three areas: in the plain of the Ganges, in the Yellow River basin, and on the Mediterranean littoral. These environments were propitious for the growth of population. They were warm enough to allow the production of sufficient foodstuff: either grain or—round the Mediterranean—olives and vines whose products could be traded for grain, yet were cool enough to inhibit the development of those infectious diseases found in tropical and equatorial regions.

In time, man creates his own environment, offering infectious diseases new opportunities. The paddyfields of China provided breeding grounds for malarial bearing mosquitos and for the transmission of schistosomiasis (see page 25) and the cities of the Roman empire provided ideal conditions for epidemic illnesses. In later times the wealth of European civilization allowed it to conquer the problems created by the process of urbanization, and the combination of wealth and a cool climate allowed these countries to develop.

The health problems of underdeveloped countries are a consequence of both their climate and their poverty, two factors which are interdependent, but whose separate contributions can be identified. If we consider some of the diseases which have occurred in Britain—cholera, hookworm, tapeworm, typhus, tetanus, smallpox, plague, malaria, typhoid, paratyphoid, and leprosy—it is obvious that many of the diseases which are today considered to be tropical diseases are, in fact, diseases of poverty. Even those diseases which could not occur in Britain because of its temperate climate can sometimes be prevented if the countries in which they are endemic only had the means to do so—trachoma, a very common cause of blindness, can be prevented by washing the face and eyes once a day with pure water (see page 37). Not all underdeveloped countries are warmer than our own. Some are colder, or drier, or both. Their real problem is that because the inhabitants are often malnourished they are prey to the infectious diseases, such as dysentery and measles, which have little effect on well-nourished inhabitants of societies which are materially more wealthy. The main cause of the inferior health of underdeveloped countries is not their climate, but under-development itself. The diseases of underdeveloped countries must be considered not only in their medical context but in the social, political, and economic context of each country. One of the most important factors in the broader context is the rate of population growth.

In March 1976 the world population was estimated to be more than 4,000 million and to be increasing by about 70 million annually. The United Nations predict that there will be 6,240 million people living on Planet Earth in the year 2,000. In India, the growth rate is 2.6 per cent per annum which, if it continues, will result in 1,000 million people in India alone by the end of the century, nearly 400 million more than at present. The population of Africa is increasing at 2.6 per cent per annum which will double population to more than 800 million by the first decade of the twenty-first century, and the population of Latin America will also double in the same period. In China the growth rate is much lower. One estimate is that it is only 1.1 per cent per annum, which is very similar to that of some developed countries, for example Canada.

By itself, population growth is a phenomenon, not a problem, but when the increase in the number of people in a country means competition for limited resources the losers suffer. In underdeveloped countries the most critical resource is food, and the most common suffering malnutrition. The Food and Agriculture Organization (F.A.O.) estimate that in 1976, 460 million people were malnourished—15 per cent of the world's population. Two-thirds of these live in South East Asia, where one-third of the population is malnourished. The main effect of malnutrition is that it increases the susceptibility to infection. It can also stunt the potential and vitiate the abilities of those who do not die of infection. They are unable to work efficiently so that they live in a vicious cycle of malnutrition and low productivity.

Vigorous attempts have been made by the World Health Organization (W.H.O.) to tackle certain diseases. Their outstanding success is the eradication of smallpox in a decade. In 1967, when W.H.O. started its campaign, smallpox affected about one million people in thirty-eight countries. By ensuring that every case was detected, and by vaccinating the contacts of each case, smallpox was eradicated in one country after another until, in 1974, only four countries—India, Pakistan, Bangladesh, and Ethiopia— suffered endemic smallpox. The final steps were hindered by war and civil unrest but the last case of smallpox was reported on 26 October 1977, except for a single case infected by virus kept in a laboratory which occured in Birmingham, England in 1978. This striking success contrasts with the more modest, yet still impressive, results of the attempts to eradicate malaria which W.H.O. started in 1958. When the programme commenced, malaria was endemic in 148 countries, but by 1975 it had been eradicated in only 37 and 1,136 million people were still at risk of infection. The programme had virtually stagnated since 1969. In comparison with smallpox, a disease spreading directly from man to man, malaria is a complex disease. The micro-organisms which cause malaria are carried by, and develop in, certain species of mosquito, those of the genus *Anopheles*, which is known as the vector of malaria. The prevention of malaria requires an attack launched simultaneously against both infected humans and vectors. This more complex biological problem requires not only wealth but a degree of public order and organization which many underdeveloped countries simply do not have. The failure of the campaign can be partly explained by biological factors, especially the development of resistant strains of malaria, but social factors have also been important. Realizing that eradication is very difficult, the emphasis of the W.H.O.

Malaria Campaign has now shifted from eradication to the control of malaria. Aware that it is not enough to reduce mortality, the W.H.O. also attacks the diseases which are not necessarily fatal but which sap the strength of the peoples of the underdeveloped world. Malaria is such a disease; trypanosomiasis—sleeping sickness—is another. The protozoa of the genus *Trypanosoma* are spread by the tsetse fly, which breeds in shade and moisture, but can adapt to open spaces. Like malaria, it can be prevented either by reducing the pool of infection by treating infected individuals, or by reducing the number of vectors, or by both methods. The problems of prevention are well illustrated by the trypanosomiasis campaign, which not only failed to eradicate the disease but did not always maintain such progress as was achieved; in 1958 only 0.02 per cent of the population of Zaire were affected, but by 1964 15 per cent were infected because the disorder of the civil war had negated the previous good efforts. Similarly, large areas of Rhodesia which had been cleared of the tsetse fly became re-infested as a result of the disruptive effects of the guerilla war on the Mozambique border.

Blindness also has serious economic consequences. At present there are 10 million blind people. The same number again have such poor vision that they are completely dependent, and the W.H.O. estimate that as many as 32 million people could be blind by 2,000 A.D. Many cases of blindness can be prevented, and the W.H.O. estimates that the number of blind people at the end of the century could be kept down to 20 million if simple preventive measures were adopted. Of the four common causes of blindness only one, cataract, clouding of the lens, offers little scope for prevention. Dietary deficiency of Vitamin A causes xerophthalmia, which is especially common in the Middle East, Central America, and South East Asia—15,000 Indian children under the age of five lose their sight every year because of this disease and 11 million children are affected world-wide. Xerophthalmia can be prevented by vitamin drops or the addition of Vitamin A to sugar. Trachoma is a viral infection which can be prevented by washing the face and eyes once a day in clean water. The fourth major cause of blindness is onchocerciasis, river blindness, infection by a filarial worm *Onchocerca volvulus*. These worms are spread by blackflies which breed in fast flowing water (hydro-electric schemes create excellent breeding grounds). Onchoceriasis affects some 20 million people in the area 15° north and south of the Equator. Although the disease was carried to the Americas by slaves it is most prevalent in Africa, especially in the Volta river basin where one person in six is affected. In some areas one-quarter of all the men over the age of thirty are blind from this disease, which can be prevented by the addition of one part of D.D.T. to one million parts of water. It was eradicated in Kenya in 1955, but remains a scourge throughout the rest of equatorial Africa.

In considering the prevention of over-population it should be emphasized that the reduction in mortality due to the prevention of disease makes only a small contribution to the increase in the world's population. The very rapid increase in recent years from 3,250 million in 1967 to 4,000 million in 1976 is due to the fact that populations naturally expand by geometric progression, unless limited by some massive check such as the Black Death. Governments have tried a wide range of solutions from education to the offer of financial rewards to encourage people to use family planning services, but only in China has there been significant success. From the 1950s Mao Tse-Tung advocated later marriage, and two children, as the norm, which encouraged the Chinese people to adopt the birth-control techniques which were simultaneously made available to them. The Chinese success is outstanding. Impotence to prevent over-population leaves many other countries no other option than to try to prevent malnutrition. The problems are daunting. Many people live in a climate in which drought is common and serious, more than 600 million people live in dry areas, and nearly 80 million people exist in deserts. To grow more food a nation requires the resources to provide irrigation and fertilizers. To keep the food which is grown it requires pesticides, storage, and distribution facilities. One-third of the milk in West Africa turns sour before it is drunk, and one-quarter of the grain produced in India rots or is eaten by vermin. These problems can be overcome, but only if sufficient finance is available and it is properly used.

The basic problem which underlies and causes disease, over-population, and malnutrition is poverty; the poverty of nations and the poverty of individuals. Poverty is the main reason why disease is much more common in underdeveloped countries, and the principal reasons why people in underdeveloped countries have many children are that they expect to lose some from the disease of poverty; they rely on children to work for them and with them; and they look to their children to provide social security in old age or illness. Malnutrition is also caused by poverty. Even where underdeveloped countries are able to produce enough food, many individuals in those countries are unable to buy enough of the food which is produced because of the social inequality which exists. A change in the structure of society will not bring down the birth-rate unaided. Family planning services are also required. Acceptable methods of birth-control and an effective distribution system; the training of paramedical staff for public education; the insertion of intra-uterine contraceptive devices; sterilization; and the availability of early out-patient termination of pregnancy are the basic measures which are required if people are to be helped to realize their wish and limit the size of their families.

A number of agencies in Britain are concerned with the stimulation of interest in such problems and in their practical solution—War On Want, Oxfam, Help the Aged, LEPRA (the British Leprosy Relief Association), Save the Children, the International Agency for the Prevention of Blindness, which is supported by the Royal Commonwealth Society for the Blind, the Churches, and many other charitable groups all serve a useful function, but the sums of money required are so great that the commitment of government is also necessary. The solution of the problems of underdeveloped countries requires aid from the developed world.

The first five year phase of the W.H.O.'s campaign against river blindness in the Volta basin will cost £60 million, an amount which would be impossible to raise in the area affected. The World Bank has focused its attention on agriculture and is now giving priority to small projects. Under the leadership of Robert McNamara the Bank, through its affiliate the International Development Association, made loans totalling $7,000 million to encourage agriculture during the period from 1974 to 1978. These figures are impressive, but two outstanding obstacles to prevention remain. The first is that these amounts are grossly inadequate: the United Nations has suggested that 0.7 per cent of each developed country's Gross National Product (G.N.P.) be allocated to overseas aid. In 1976 only three of the seventeen richest countries—Sweden,

Holland, and Norway—reached this target. The United States made the least sacrifice at 0.26 per cent of its G.N.P., and in 1978 Congress cut 13 per cent from the contribution to the International Development Association on the recommendation of President Carter; the United Kingdom gave only 0.34 per cent of its G.N.P. The OPEC countries give more than 3 per cent of their G.N.P. to aid underdeveloped countries. Susan George, in her excellent analysis of the causes of world poverty and hunger, *How The Other Half Dies*, estimates that the increased price of oil to underdeveloped countries has been more than met by the increased aid given them by OPEC and makes it clear where the responsibility for aid lies in the developed world. In 1978 Britain took a significant step by cancelling over £900 million of debts from twenty poor countries, which will cost about £60 million annually in lost interest, and other developed countries also published plans to cancel debts. Much more could still be done by the developed world. The second, and more intractable, problem lies in the political and economic structure of underdeveloped countries. Any aid given may be used by a small proportion of the population for its own benefit, not only by the retention of funds but by encouraging the development of cash crops for export rather than food crops for consumption. Although exports create wealth, the wealth again returns to only a small proportion of the population, the landholders, leaving the majority impoverished and unable to buy enough of that food which is produced.

The underdeveloped countries are very different from one another. No general solution is applicable to them all, but one principle appears to be valid and relevant in every case. The prevention of over-population, disease, and malnutrition requires not only a redistribution of wealth from the rich, developed countries to those which are underdeveloped but also a redistribution of wealth and the means of creating wealth—land—within the underdeveloped countries themselves.

Within almost every underdeveloped country, however, much disease could be prevented by making better use of resources, without major changes in social economic structures. By the careful selection of common, serious, preventable diseases as health care priorities, the use of cheaper, less highly-trained auxiliaries wherever possible, and the development of community-based services rather than those centred on hospitals, more effective and efficient use of resources can be made. In addition to financial aid technical help is also given by developed countries, for example by the Ministry of Overseas Development, but for that technical advice to be taken requires the right approach in the underdeveloped country to which it is given. *Medical Care in Developing Countries—A Primer on the Medicine of Poverty* edited by Maurice King, and *Primary Child Care* by Maurice and Felicity King and Soebagio Martodipoero, both textbooks for underdeveloped countries, give an excellent illustration of the requisite approach, which has to take into account not only scientific theory but also the culture in which that theory has to be put into practice.

4   The promotion of child health

Prevention of genetic and chromosomal disorders

Each human cell contains forty-six chromosomes. Forty-four are called autosomes, being similar in both sexes and consisting of twenty-two pairs. The other two are the sex chromosomes: in men an X and a Y chromosome, in women two X chromosomes. In the testis and ovary, cells divide producing not identical cells with forty-six chromosomes, as in other tissues of the body during the normal process of cell division, but cells with twenty-three chromosomes; the reproductive gametes. In the testis are formed spermatozoa, half of which have twenty-two autosomes and an X chromosome, the other half having twenty-two autosomes and a Y chromosome. In the ovary are formed ova, all of which have twenty-two chromosomes and an X chromosome so that, at conception, a forty-six chromosome cell is formed by fusion of the male and female gametes.

Each chromosome is a chain of genes. Each gene is located at a fixed site or *locus*, and the sequence of genes is the same on both chromosomes in each pair of autosomes. The pair of genes may or may not be identical. For example, at the ABO blood group *locus* on the relevant pair of chromosomes any two out ot the three possible genes A, B, or O may be present. A and B are dominant genes, O is recessive, so that if the gene pair is B and O the person's blood will be group B, just as if the pair of genes inherited were B and B. Genes A and B are equally dominant so that someone who inherits A from one parent and B from another will have blood group AB and a person will only be blood group O if both his genes are O. Each gene contains information coded by the sequence of chemical units which compose it and programme the cell to function in a certain way. The numerous genes which determine height or hair colour are relatively unimportant, but some genes contain vital information. For example, one gene contains the information necessary to make a protein essential for blood clotting. If it is missing, the person's blood fails to clot, with disastrous results: this is the cause of haemophilia (see page 33). Some harmful genes are dominant—that is a child need only inherit one to be affected—others are recessive. People who carry one recessive gene are not impaired, but they are called carriers. If two carriers marry, their children may receive a pair of recessive genes and be affected.

It is known with certainty that there are over 1,500 single gene disorders and another 1,000 conditions may be caused in the same way. The most common single gene disorder in Britain is cystic fibrosis in which the lung and gut secretions are chemically abnormal, resulting in lung infection and the inability to absorb food. This occurs about once in every 2,000 births. Although cystic fibrosis and all other such disorders are uncommon, they are of importance not only to the individual families affected but to the community, because they cause much of the mortality and handicap in children in developed countries. As the scourge of infectious disease is reduced, genetic disorders become relatively more important until they are more common than infection as a cause of childhood illness, handicap, and death. But it should be emphasized that underdeveloped countries are not free from genetic disorders even though the common causes of death are malnutrition and infection. In parts of Africa thousands of children die every year from sickle cell anaemia, a disorder caused by a single abnormal gene which results in abnormal haemoglobin, the oxygen-carrying blood pigment. In Thailand alone about 400,000 children are chronically ill from thalassaemia, another genetic disorder which results in abnormal haemoglobin formation. Both these diseases have become more common in Britain as the number of immigrants has increased.

Single gene disorders can be prevented by genetic counselling (see page 47) but disorders which are the result of an inheritance of a number of genes are more difficult to prevent. Congenital heart disease and congenital dislocation of the hips are two conditions which occur in greater frequency in the relatives of an affected child than they occur in the general population, indicating that genetic factors are implicated, but it is probable that the genetic inheritance does not cause the disorder directly, as is the case with cystic fibrosis. It seems that it predisposes the foetus to the development of the condition of certain environmental factors that are present. For example, the inheritance of a number of genes which make the joints a little more lax than usual will predispose a foetus to hip dislocation if, by chance, it happens to be in the breech position in the uterus. Such disorders are difficult to prevent but their effects can be mitigated by the early diagnosis and treatment of these conditions. A good example of this approach is the prevention of the effects of phenylketonuria (P.K.U.), a disorder affecting about sixty children a year in which the children are unable to metabolize certain proteins and become mentally handicapped if they eat them. The diagnosis can be made on a drop of blood drawn from the baby's heel and the parents can then be helped to provide the special diet necessary to prevent handicap.

Other handicaps are due to disorders of whole chromosomes. During the process of cell division in the ovary and testis, gametes are sometimes formed which have 23 autosomes and one sex chromosome instead of the normal complement of 22 autosomes and one sex chromosome. If an ovum with 24 chromosomes is fertilized by a normal sperm with 23 chromosomes, the resulting foetus, if it survives, will have 47 chromosomes—45 chromosomes together with two sex chromosomes. The disorder which results depends from which particular pair of autosomes the extra chromosome derives. If it is from the pair of autosomes numbered 21 in autosome classification, the result is mongolism, now called Down's syndrome. Down's syndrome is an important cause of severe mental handicap and about one-third of all mentally-handicapped children are affected by this condition. It occurs once in every 600 births, that is about 1,000 affected babies are born in England and Wales every year. In 1970 nearly 17 per cent of the births of infant's with Down's syndrome were born to the 2 per cent of mothers aged over 40 and another 18 per cent were born to the 6 per cent of mothers aged between 35 and 39. (The frequency of the syndrome increases rapidly with age, increasing from one in 1,000 in women less than 30 years old to one in sixty in women aged over 45.)

There is scope for the prevention of Down's syndrome by ensuring that all older women are aware of the greatly increased risk, and are offered an appropriate method of family planning. Some older women still become pregnant unaware of the risk whilst others know of and accept it; but pregnant women who are at risk can now be informed at ante-natal clinics and offered the opportunity of a test to see whether or not the foetus they are carrying is abnormal. The test consists of the microscopic examination of the chromosomes of foetal cells obtained by aspirating a sample of the amniotic fluid which surrounds the foetus, the sample being obtained by inserting a long needle through the lower abdominal wall into the uterine cavity. This procedure, amniocentesis, is not without risk to the foetus, so the parents' decision whether or not to accept the opportunity of amniocentesis can be very difficult. They have to consider not only the secondary decision of whether or not to request an abortion if the foetus is abnormal, but the possibility of losing, through an induced abortion caused by a procedure agreed to by themselves, a normal foetus. Because amniocentesis facilities are expensive and because there is a risk to the normal foetus, the opportunity is usually offered only to older women. From which age the test should be offered is a matter of opinion. The lower the ages of women offered the test, the greater will be the cost per case detected as the higher will be the proportion of women tested who are carrying normal foetuses.

Most people consider that the service should be offered to women over forty and many say that all pregnant women over the age of thirty-five should be included. Even if all women over the age of thirty-five were offered, and accepted, amniocentesis, many handicapped children (about 400 per year) would still be born to younger women, but some of these births could also be prevented. The great majority of cases of Down's syndrome are born to normal parents one of whom—usually the mother—happens to have formed an abnormal gamete with an extra chromosome. A small proportion, about two per cent, are born to parents one of whom has an abnormal complement of chromosomes in all their cells although he or she appears to be normal. Parents who are liable to conceive another affected baby can now be identified by the analysis of parental chromosomes and parents can then be counselled about the risk of recurrence.

Amniocentesis also plays a key part in the prevention of spina bifida. Nervous tissue develops from a flat area of embryonic cells. In the normal foetus two ridges of cells form which meet to form a closed tube of nervous tissue, a part of which exposes to become the brain, the remainder becoming the spinal cord. In about one in 350 foetuses, this process is imperfect. If the tube of nervous tissue does not close completely this results in anencephaly if the defect was at the brain end of the tube, or a baby may be born with a defect in the spinal cord; this is spina bifida, which occurs about once in every 500 births, and nervous tissue is open to the skin instead of being a closed tube inside the bony vertebral canal. The child is often paralyzed below the level of the spinal cord defect and there is sometimes associated hydrocephalus—increased fluid pressure inside the brain—which can cause mental deficiency. A blood test has been developed to detect those pregnant women who are at high risk of carrying a foetus with spina bifida. From the flat area of embryonic nervous tissue formed in all foetuses, a specific protein called alphafeto-protein leaks from the embryonic nerve cells into the fluid surrounding the foetus and then across the placenta into the mother's blood stream. Alphafeto-protein can therefore be detected in the blood stream of all pregnant women, but the level of this protein normally decreases as the flat area of nervous tissue grows to form the closed tube of nervous tissue. If the foetus has spina bifida, however, the level of protein does not decrease. Unfortunately, it is not possible to discriminate between the normal and abnormal results with complete certainty because the blood levels in a small proportion of women who are carrying normal foetuses is higher than the level in a small proportion of those women who are carrying a foetus with spina bifida. One approach is to offer further tests to the three per cent of women with the highest blood levels of alphafeto protein. Ultrasonic scan can detect those women who are carrying twins, a normal cause of high levels of alphafeto protein, and locate the position of the placenta, the site at which the foetal umbilical cord is attached to the uterus, which allows the obstetrician to perform an amniocentesis with less risk to the foetus. Measurement of the alphafeto-protein level of the amniotic fluid withdrawn allows the diagnosis of spina bifida to be made with certainty, and the parents can be offered an abortion. By this procedure more than eighty per cent of those of foetuses which have spina bifida can be detected. In the other twenty per cent of cases the alphafeto-protein level is below the level chosen to distinguish the three per cent who are offered amniocentesis from the ninety-seven per cent who are not. The proportion of cases could be increased by lowering the arbitrary level, for example by conducting spinal examinations including amniocentesis on the ten per cent with the highest levels. This would, however, expose many more pregnant women with normal foetuses to the small risk entailed in amniocentesis.

To summarize: if 1,000 women receive the blood test, those thirty who have the highest levels will have a second blood test. At this second blood test about half will have levels which are undoubtedly normal so they can be reassured. This leaves fifteen for ultrasonography and amniocentesis of whom two will have an affected foetus. The procedure has been made to sound simple, but the prevention of spina bifida and other genetic disorders bristles with ethical problems. Many people find the abortion of handicapped foetuses no easier to accept than the abortion of normal foetuses. There are also practical problems, notably the cost of these preventive services (see page 154).

At all stages of the procedures designed to prevent the birth of bodies affected by genetic disorders, chromosomal disorder such as Down's syndrome, and spina bifida, sound and sympathetic counsel is necessary for parents faced by harrowing options, but there are only less than thirty centres in Britain at which expert genetic counselling is available. Genetic counselling, valuable though it is, only prevents the birth of handicapped babies by precluding their conception and by facilitating the abortion of those already handicapped. Another aspect is the prevention of damage to normal foetuses while they are developing in the uterus and while they are being born.

Prevention in pregnancy and labour

The placenta is the site at which the foetal umbilical cord is attached to the uterus. The maternal blood vessels which run to and from the uterus divide into a network of small vessels, as do the umbilical blood vessels of the foetus. The mother's blood never mixes with that of the foetus, but in the placenta the two blood streams are separated only by a thin layer of cells across which diffuse oxygen and other nutrients, from mother to foetus, and waste products which require excretion, from foetus to mother.

Across this thin layer bacteria and viruses can also pass, some of which can damage the foetus. Syphilis used to be a common cause of congenital handicap but congenital syphilis has now been virtually eradicated. Penicillin cures syphilis, so women who catch the disease can be cleared of infection in a short period of time and the probability of a woman with syphilis becoming pregnant is now remote. Should that occur, however, the syphilis will be diagnosed because every pregnant woman is tested for syphilis at an early stage in pregnancy when an abortion is simple to perform. Syphilis affects adults severely—it can be fatal—so its serious effects on a foetus are not surprising. German measles, infection by the rubella virus, is usually mild in adults but it can cause severe mental and physical handicap in the baby if a pregnant woman is infected. This was first reported in 1941 by an Australian ophthalmologist who was struck by a sudden increase in the number of babies who had congenital cataract—clouding of the lens of the eye. He investigated these cases in detail and found that the mothers had had rubella during pregnancy. His first tentative conclusions were soon confirmed and the passage of rubella virus across the placenta from mother to foetus was found to be a cause of a number of congenital defects, of which the commonest are cataract, brain damage, deafness, and congenital heart disease—occurring singly or in combination. It took almost thirty years to develop a rubella vaccine, but in 1970 this became available and the school health service began to vaccinate girls of about twelve years of age. The immunity which vaccination stimulates renders these girls resistant to rubella infection so that if they should have contact with an infected child or adult in later life, when pregnant, the virus will neither enter their bloodstream nor damage their foetus. It is impossible to say how many handicaps will be prevented by this policy because it has never been possible to determine precisely how many babies were congenitally handicapped by rubella.

Even if all women of child-bearing age have been made immune by vaccination, handicap would probably be prevented in one thousand babies each year, an extremely important contribution. Two other infectious diseases, toxoplasmosis and cytomegalovirus infection, also cause foetal damage although the infected pregnant woman, like other adults, rarely experiences severe symptoms.

Research to produce vaccines against these micro-organisms is in progress but the number of babies who would benefit is unknown, and the risks which might be associated with such vaccinations are also uncertain.

Not only living micro-organisms pass from the mother into the foetus; some chemicals pass across the placenta with harmful effects. The most dramatic example of this was provided by thalidomide. Introduced by standards which were thought to be adequate and prescribed by well-intentioned doctors to bring sleep to tired pregnant women, the chemical affected the foetal limb buds at a crucial stage in their development, with the result that limbless babies were born. The repercussions of the thalidomide tragedy have been far-reaching. Society and government took a fresh look at the principle of liability and compensation (see page 15) and medicine and the pharmaceutical industry reviewed the way in which they developed, tested, and introduced new drugs. A Medicines Act was placed on the Statute Book in 1968 and a statutory Committee on Safety of Medicines was instituted in 1970 to reduce the risk of drugs with harmful side-effects being put on the market. Medical and public education has since attempted to dissuade doctors and lay people from the use of any sort of drug in pregnancy unless it is absolutely necessary, so some good has come from the tragedy. The foetus is at risk from other chemicals. Alcohol can damage the foetus if taken excessively and the babies of alcoholic women who have continued to drink throughout pregnancy may be handicapped, suffering from a combination of different impairments which are together known as the foetal alcohol syndrome; but there is as yet no evidence that social drinking affects foetal development. It now seems certain that blighted potatoes and soft water do not cause foetal malformation, but the risks associated with industrial pollution are an area of uncertainty. The risk lies not only in the accidental release of substances known to be toxic. Each new process produces many by-products of uncertain properties (see page 173) some of which may be harmful to foetuses if the by-product is inhaled or ingested by pregnant women. One particularly dangerous type of product is radioactive material. The dangers to the foetus of X-raying pregnant women are well-known and doctors now avoid such investigations during pregnancy wherever possible, although the increasing amount of

radioactive material in all developed countries has serious implications for the future because radioactivity can affect not only a
normal developing foetus but also the cells in testis and ovary
causing genetic and chromosomal abnormalities in sperms and
ova, resulting in the conception of abnormal foetuses.

Harmful chemicals may be produced by the mother herself.
People with diabetes produce abnormally high levels of normal
body chemicals and these can affect foetal development. Still
births and other complications of pregnancy are more common in
women who are diabetic, but they can be prevented by careful
control of the diabetes together with the induction of labour before
the full period of gestation has expired, although this is only
undertaken with reluctance. Prematurity puts the new-born baby
at risk (see page 53), but there comes a point in the pregnancy of
diabetic women, usually between the thirty-sixth and thirty-eighth
week, when the risk of prematurity may be less than the risk of
allowing the pregnancy to continue to its full forty-week duration,
because the risks to the foetus of a diabetic woman increase quickly
in the last few weeks of pregnancy.

Not only simple molecules, like glucose, pass from mother to
foetus; more complex molecules, such as proteins, can pass through
the cells of the placenta. Antibodies are proteins and they pass into
the foetal bloodstream with the result that the new-born baby has
some immunity against infection, although the most effective means
of transferring immunity is breast-feeding. One type of antibody,
the rhesus antibody, is, however, harmful and can cause handicap
and death. People who have 'rhesus positive' blood have a certain
protein in their blood which is absent from 'rhesus negative' blood.
Those who are rhesus positive have either one or two rhesus genes,
which are dominant (see page 42), and it is only people who have
no rhesus genes who are rhesus negative. A rhesus negative mother
will conceive a rhesus positive foetus if the successful sperm contains
a rhesus gene from the father. The first such pregnancy is unevent-
ful for the foetus but it sometimes happens that a small amount of
foetal blood passes into the mother's bloodstream while the placenta
is separating from the uterus after birth or abortion. If this happens,
the rhesus negative mother may make antibodies against the rhesus
protein in the blood of her rhesus positive child. If she should
subsequently conceive another rhesus positive foetus, these

antibodies, formed in response to the blood of the first foetus, can pass from mother to foetus during pregnancy and destroy the foetal blood cells, causing anaemia and jaundice, which may result in brain damage or death of the foetus. This disorder is called rhesus haemolytic disease because the destruction of red blood cells is a process termed haemolysis.

A number of effective measures have been developed which have prevented stillbirths, infant death, and mental handicap resulting from this condition. Routine blood tests of all pregnant women reveal those at risk—those who are rhesus negative, especially those in whom the rhesus antibody can be detected. Such women are closely supervised during pregnancy and if the level of antibody rises too much, premature induction of labour is considered, although the benefits of this step have to be weighed against the risks of prematurity (see page 53). It is now possible to give the foetus a blood transfusion while it is still in the uterus to allow the pregnancy to continue for a further period. After birth the newborn jaundiced baby requires special care. Sometimes the exchange transfusion of blood is undertaken by the removal of its blood, with the damaged red cells, and the simultaneous transfusion of donor blood free from antibodies into another part of its circulatory system. These measures have all been designed to minimize the effects of rhesus antibody on the growing foetus but the development of a new technique now allows the prevention of the formation of the antibody in the first place. If a rhesus negative woman is injected with rhesus antibody immediately after delivery of a rhesus positive baby, the injected antibody destroys any foetal red cells which might have leaked from the placenta into the mother's bloodstream before they can stimulate her to form rhesus antibodies.

Between 1968 and 1975 the stillbirth rate (the number of stillbirths per thousand births) fell from 0.52 to 0.16, a decrease from 430 still births to 100. During the same period the infant mortality rate (the number of infants under the age of one year dying per thousand live births) fell from 0.19 to 0.06, a decrease from 158 to 36 post-natal deaths. Although precise figures do not exist, it can be assumed that the number of babies surviving with brain damage fell at a corresponding rate. The prevention of rhesus haemolytic disease highlights the role of obstetricians in prevention and emphasizes once more that the preventive approach and the use of high technology are often closely interrelated.

At no time is the risk of death and brain damage as high as at birth and in the week following. The risk to the mother has been greatly decreased by antibiotics and blood transfusion and by more careful antenatal supervision. The child is much less at risk now compared with one hundred years or more ago when many children died as a result of obstetric procedures or infection, but many preventable deaths and handicaps still occur. The main risk factor is now low birth weight. Not all babies need necessarily weigh the same. There is a normal range of birth weights and some babies weigh much less than the average without showing any ill effects. In general, however, babies which are lighter are more at risk of dying or being handicapped. Seven per cent of babies weigh less than 2,500 G (5.5 lbs) and one per cent weigh less than 1,500 G (3.3 lbs) at birth, and it is these groups who are most at risk. It should be emphasized that babies cannot be classified into distinct groups—the lighter the baby the greater the risk of death or handicap—but of those weighing less than 1,500 G at birth only forty per cent survive the first year of life, and half of them have some defect which was caused by brain damage at or immediately after delivery. The new-born baby is immature in very many ways and the lower the weight the less the maturity. The baby of low birth weight is unable to maintain its body temperature. The control of its energy balance and other metabolic functions are less well developed and its lungs are not completely adapted to take in oxygen. A drop in body temperature, or in the concentration of blood glucose or oxygen, can cause brain damage which results in mental handicap and spastic paralysis—sometimes called cerebral palsy—and these are more common if the birth weight is low.

The birth weight is determined by many factors, some of which are genetic. Some foetuses have a greater potential for gaining weight than others, but whether or not the foetus achieves its genetic potential depends principally on two factors; the adequacy of the nutrition from its mother through the placenta while it is in the uterus, and the length of time it spends there. The average duration of pregnancy is 280 days, although normal pregnancy can be a few days longer or a few days less. If, however, the baby is born before it has completed its full period of intra-uterine growth it will not have achieved its full potential weight. Such an early baby has a low birth weight. The earlier the baby, the lower the birth weight and the greater the risk of death and brain damage. Not surprisingly, spontaneous early onset of labour is more common in twin pregnancies, but in single pregnancies the cause is often unknown and therefore impossible to prevent. Sometimes doctors 'cause' low birth weight babies by inducing labour early if they think that the risks of early delivery are less than the risks to the foetus of maternal diabetes or rhesus antibodies (see page 50). The careful management of diabetes and the prevention of the development of rhesus antibodies can therefore preclude the need for induction of labour, and so prevent some babies being born early.

In developed countries the state of nutrition of pregnant women is usually adequate to supply the foetus with all its requirements. Foetal malnutrition only rarely occurs as a result of maternal malnutrition, as commonly occurs in underdeveloped countries. It is more usually due to a placental deficiency. The most common causes of placental deficiency are those diseases which affect the maternal blood vessels—high blood pressure and pre-eclamptic toxaemia—and the effects of cigarette smoke are similar. Still birth and death in the first week of life is nearly thirty per cent more common in the babies of women who smoke regularly after the fourth month of pregnancy. The main reason for this is that the babies are smaller at birth; the baby of a woman who smokes is on average 150 to 250 G (5 to 9 oz.) lighter than that of a non-smoker. It has been estimated that as many as 1,500 babies die each year, and that many more are handicapped by the effects of cigarette smoke. The actual mechanism by which the chemicals of tobacco smoke cause damage is uncertain but the most probable is the effect of the smoke on those maternal blood vessels which supply the placenta.

Babies whose birth weight is low because of starvation in the uterus are sometimes called growth retarded to distinguish them from early babies, but the two conditions can occur together. The early onset of labour can occur in a pregnancy in which the foetus is being starved, just as it can occur in a normal pregnancy, and in such cases prematurity and growth retardation are coincidental. In other cases the two conditions occur together because the obstetrician decided on an early induction of labour by artificial means to prevent the effects of placental deficiency, which are greatest in the last few weeks of pregnancy when the foetus is biggest and most demanding. If the baby remains in the uterus much longer than 280 days it may also be affected as the placenta becomes progressively inefficient after the normal duration of pregnancy has been passed.

Two approaches are possible to prevent the mortality and handicap which more commonly affect babies of low birth weight— the prevention of low birth weight itself, and the provision of more effective services for the care of early and growth retarded babies in the neonatal period immediately after birth.

Specific measures to prevent the early onset of labour are difficult to develop because the basic cause is known in only a small proportion of cases. An indirect approach is through the better management of rhesus disease and diabetes which can preclude the need for artificial induction before the full duration of pregnancy has expired. The primary prevention of pre-eclampsic toxaemia and high blood pressure is not possible at present but their effects can be mitigated by the prevention of obesity and by ensuring adequate rest for affected women. Not only does the control of high blood pressure in pre-eclampsia improve the nutrition of the foetus but it allows the doctor supervising the pregnancy to postpone the induction of labour until the estimated date of delivery if he remains satisfied that the foetus is growing at an adequate rate. Thus such simple measures as rest and the prevention of obesity can prevent placental problems, the need to induce labour arti- ficially (a procedure which sometimes eventually requires deli- very by caesarean section), early delivery, low birth weight, brain damage, and death. However, these simple measures are not always easy to implement—nor is the prevention of cigarette smoking in pregnancy easy to achieve. The cigarette consump- tion of pregnant women has reduced but tobacco still causes many deaths and handicaps. The problem of cigarette smoking in pregnancy has to be considered in the broader context of its prevention (see page 160).

Because the primary causes of low birth-weight are difficult to prevent it is, and always will be, necessary to provide services for the support of low birth-weight babies but there is evidence to suggest that the services in Britain have not improved as much as those of other countries, for example France. In 1960 the infant mortality rate—the number of babies dying in their first year per 1,000 live births—was twenty-two per cent higher in France than in Britain. A decade later the French rate was ten per cent lower and, as infant mortality rate is a dependable indicator of the health of young children, it could be concluded that the proportion of children who are handicapped in France is now less than in Britain. During this decade of progress France invested resources in both buildings and manpower to improve the services for low birth weight babies. There is no doubt that the provision of special care baby units is better in some regions of Britain than in others, and one solution would be to provide money, buildings, and equipment in regions which are less well served. Another solution would be to identify just which factors within the range of skills and services concentrated in special care baby units are the critical ones, and to provide them in all obstetric hospitals. One factor which seems to be of particular importance is the skill of medical staff who have specialized in neonatal paediatrics in emergency resuscitation. This would not of course preclude the need for special care baby units.

The answer does not only lie in the provision of more resources. More effective use could perhaps be made of those resources at present available. This does not mean that resources should all be diverted to one style of obstetric care: the future use of resources cannot be set out in a series of simple questions such as the comparative merits of home and hospital delivery, or whether babies should be delivered in general practitioner obstetric units, or wards supervised by consultant obstetricians, or in teaching hospitals. A range of services, including delivery at home, G.P. units, consultant units in non-teaching hospitals, and professorial units in teaching hospitals will continue to be provided in the future as they are at present, but more effective use of these could be made without extensive reorganization.

There are still women and babies at risk who are not referred to a more specialized service at the appropriate time. General practitioner units, for example, are safe provided that cases at high risk are referred to a consultant or professorial unit either during the antenatal period, or during labour if the risk only becomes manifest at that stage. The unexpected will always occur in obstetrics, but many complications can be anticipated if doctors are alert and work in close co-operation with those in different branches of the obstetric service.

The training of obstetricians, paediatricians, and general practitioners has improved greatly in recent years. They make better use of the range of services than they did formerly, referring women at risk to a more appropriate service soon enough for that service to minimize the risk, but education of the patients has proved more difficult. The perinatal mortality rate, the number of still births and deaths in the first week of life per thousand total births, still varies very much, from 7.5 per 1,000 in social class II to 27.6 per 1,000 in social class V (see page 153). There are many reasons for this, but the main preventable factor is the different use of the available services.

Women in social class V go to clinic for the first time later in the course of pregnancy, attend less regularly, and follow the advice given less punctiliously. For instance, they more frequently continue to smoke. There may be sound practical reasons for these differences. A mother of three, married to a man whose earnings are low, depending on public transport, may find it more difficult to reach the antenatal clinic than the wife of a doctor with one child and her own car, but there are also social reasons (see page 143). In France the problem of poor clinic attendance was largely solved by paying a financial benefit which was contingent on regular clinic attendance, and the same approach may be needed in Britain if those people most at risk are to be seen at clinics early and often enough, and if it is thought to be ethically acceptable. The prevention of problems in pregnancy and labour requires an approach which considers not only the medical skills required but the attitudes and aspirations of pregnant women and their husbands, which are influenced by their social and economic background.

Prevention in childhood

Although the first health visiting service was started by the Manchester and Salford Ladies Sanitary Reform Association in 1867, and the first school medical officer was appointed by the London School Board in 1890, it was not until the first decade of the twentieth century that the full extent of childhood handicap and mortality was recognized and tackled by government intervention (see page 13). The decrease in mortality since then has been striking.

Mortality in childhood in England and Wales (the figures for children under 1 year old are the number of deaths per year per 1000 live births; the figures for older age groups are the number of deaths per year per 1000 children of that age)

	Under 1	1–4	5–9	10–14	15–19
1911	130.1	17.7	3.4	2.1	2.9
1931	66.4	7.6	2.1	1.5	2.5
1951	29.7	1.4	0.6	0.5	0.8
1974	16.3	0.7	0.3	0.3	0.6

Source: *Fit for the Future*, The Report of the Committee on Child Health Services, Cmnd. 6684, H.M.S.O., 1976, p.41.

Most of this decline is due to a decrease in the mortality from the common infectious diseases resulting principally from improvements in nutrition, the introduction of vaccination (see page 10), the development of antibiotics, and a natural decline in the severity of some infections (see page 4).

Deaths of children in England and Wales

| | 1911–15 | | 1970–74 | |
	Number	Deaths per million	Number	Deaths per million
Pneumonia & bronchitis	76,643	1,464	2,330	43
Tuberculosis	46,459	887	71	1
Diphtheria	23,380	447	1	0
Accidents	18,500	353	7,214	133
Measles	48,986	936	111	2
Whooping cough (Pertussis)	20,182	385	7	0
Gastroenteritis	25,560	488	487	9
Appendicitis	3,997	76	151	3
Cancer	2,388	46	3,743	69
Disease of the ear	2,515	48	59	1
Scarlet fever	9,901	189	0	0
Rheumatic fever	3,498	67	6	0

The figures for rheumatic fever are not strictly comparable because of revision of disease classification.
Source: *Fit for the Future*, The Report of the Committee on Child Health Services, Cmnd. 6684, H.M.S.O., 1976, p.41

The common causes of death are now accidents, many of which are preventable (see page 82), and various types of cancer which are, unfortunately, not preventable, but the emphasis in child health this century has been just as much on the prevention of disability and handicap as on the prevention of premature death, and the health of children shows many other signs of improvement. During the last seventy years the average height of children aged between 5 and 7 has increased by between 1 and 2 cm. each decade, and the average height of children aged from 10–14 years has increased by between 2 and 3 cm. each decade. Although obesity has become a problem, the increased height and weight of children reflects their better nutrition which has fortified their resistance to infectious diseases.

This century has seen the decline of many of the crippling diseases which affected Edwardian children. In 1914 the school health service report stated that 'between half and one per cent of the children of school age are in greater or less degree disabled by crippling disease. The chief cause is tuberculosis.' In Birmingham in 1910, for example, 128 out of 212 children in special schools suffered from tuberculosis of the spine, hip, and other joints. This disease is now a very rare cause of disability. Polio (infantile paralysis) was also a common cause of disability, but is now rare. In a survey in Edinburgh in 1903, forty-two per cent of children were found to have defective hearing and thirty-one per cent had defective vision. There are still deaf and blind children, but the use of antibiotics in the treatment of bacterial infections of the nose, throat, and ears now prevents the terrible suppurating conditions of the mastoid and middle ear, and the visual testing of all children allows the detection and correction of squints and refractive errors. Rickets was once a common disabling and disfiguring disease among British children. However, the clearing of smoke from the air and the provision of more play space allows children to receive more ultraviolet light from the sun to manufacture their own Vitamin D. This, together with the provision of cod liver oil and other Vitamin D preparations to mothers of young children, the greater availability of milk, and the addition of Vitamin D to certain foods, has virtually eradicated rickets, except in immigrant children whose skin pigment blocks the ultraviolet light so they cannot manufacture Vitamin D in the weak British sunlight, and whose diets sometimes contain insufficient vitamin to make good this deficiency.

Any changes which might have taken place in the number of children who are mentally handicapped are difficult to calculate because the definition of educational subnormality has changed over the years. In January 1977 more than 191,000 pupils, about 1.8 per cent of the school population in Britain, were attending special schools and classes for handicapped children for the whole of their education. In addition about 500,000 pupils, another five per cent of the school population, were attending special classes for some of their education, and it has been estimated that a further eight per cent of school children would, in the opinion of their teachers, benefit from such help if it were available. The Committee of Enquiry into the Education of Handicapped Children and Young People—the Warnock Report (Cmnd. 7212 H.M.S.O. 1978)—recommended that the planning of services for children and young people should be based on the assumption that one in six children will require some form of special educational provision. The common causes of handicap are no longer physical diseases but intellectual retardation and psychiatric disorder. Intellectual retardation, sometimes called mental subnormality or handicap, may be caused by brain damage, but it may also be caused by the social conditions in which a child is reared.

Material deprivation is still common in Britain, as the National Child Development Study revealed. This Study has followed the development of 10,504 children who were born in the first week of March 1958; only a very few children born in that week have not been kept under surveillance. In 1969 when the children were eleven years old, information was obtained about their social, educational, and medical circumstances which revealed a depressing pattern of deprivation. Fourteen per cent of children lived in families in which the income was below the qualifying level for supplementary benefit or free school meals. This amounts to two million children. Eighteen per cent of children were living in a house which was over-crowded, that is, it had more than 1½ persons per room; a stringent criterion as a mother, father, and four children occupying a living room, kitchen, and two bedrooms are not statutorily over-crowded. Nine per cent were living in housing which lacked hot water. The total number of children living in such conditions at some time during their schooling was calculated to be three and a half million.

These findings refer, of course, to groups and not to individual children. There are many examples of children in large, single-parent, poor, or badly housed families who thrive and succeed, but for the majority these conditions impose a social handicap on development, especially when more than one factor affects the child. One child in every sixteen was growing up in a large or single-parent family which was poor and badly housed, although this proportion varied very much from one part of Britain to another. In the south of England only one child in forty-seven was in this category, in Wales and northern England the proportion was one in twelve, and in Scotland it was one child in ten. In Northern Ireland, which was not included in the study, it was, and is, probably even higher.

As a result of the deficiencies of antenatal care, one in twelve of the disadvantaged children weighed less than 2,500G (5.5 lbs) at birth, compared with one in twenty of the children who were not disadvantaged. Those socially handicapped were shorter in height, more often absent from school, more frequently had hearing loss, more often had a squint, and were twice as likely to have had tuberculosis, meningitis, or rheumatic fever. Their housing conditions made both the spread of infectious disease more probable and accidents more common; one in seven of the disadvantaged group had suffered a burn or scald, compared with one in eleven of children not socially disadvantaged. The parents of disadvantaged children made less use of available health services, antenatal clinics, child health clinics, and immunization services. Not surprisingly, the educational achievement of deprived children was lower. One in fourteen of the disadvantaged children was receiving, or waiting to receive, special education, compared with one in eighty of those not socially handicapped, and educational subnormality was seven times more common.

Material deprivation is not new; it was even more common in the past, but the new aspect of social disadvantage is that children experience it unsupported by a stable social network. In the past poverty, bad housing, and large families were common but both nuclear and extended families were close and supportive and the values of working-class life were relatively stable. Since the Divorce

Reform Act of 1969 the divorce rate has increased—over 100,000 marriages a year now end in divorce—leaving many children in single-parent families. Divorce divides the family. It may separate the mother from her parents and the child from his grandparents. Stable communities break down as people move and values change at an increasing rate. These social changes have their effects on children, and emotional, cognitive, and existential disorders, which cause problems of learning and behaviour, are becoming increasingly common in all social classes. Children not only suffer parental deprivation more frequently—they also suffer parental assault in increasing numbers. One estimate is that more than 5,000 children are injured every year, of whom 1,000 are seriously injured and nearly 100 die.

Recognizing that the existing pattern of professional services was shaped by problems which were no longer common, the Department of Health and Social Security and the Department of Education and Science, together with the Welsh Office, convened a Committee to review the child health services, to judge how effective they were, and to propose objectives, organization, and staffing for a new integrated child health service. The Report of the Court Committee, so-called after the Chairman, a professor of paediatrics, discussed the changing pattern of child health and disease, the needs of particular groups, such as adolescents and children who were psychiatrically disordered, and the changes they saw as being necessary. Among the many stimulating recommendations was the call for specialized 'general practitioner paediatricians', 'child health visitors', and 'consultant community paediatricians'; the consideration of adolescents as a distinct group requiring specialized health services; the fluoridation of water supplies; and the need for special Parliamentary Reports on services for children. These, and the many other recommendations, suggested that a fundamental reshaping of the child health services with an emphasis on prevention was necessary.

The measures necessary to prevent the medical causes of death, disability, and handicap have been described. There are practical, ethical, and financial constraints, but the opportunities for prevention are clear to see in comparison with the prevention of social disadvantages and handicap. Simple attempts to solve housing problems by the creation of new estates and towns have had no more than moderate success, and include some dreadful failures. The mitigation of family poverty has been hindered by national poverty and a lack of political sympathy with the plight of disadvantaged families. The birth-rate has fallen, as has the average completed family size, but there is evidence that the family planning services have not reached those whose families would benefit most. A direct attack on these social problems by the provision of more professional services is necessary, but it cannot succeed in isolation. The problems have to be tackled in their political and economic contexts.

5 Prevention in adult life

Prevention of premature death

In developed countries the expectation of life of male babies at
birth is, on average, about seventy years; that of female babies is
nearly seventy-five years. The expectation of life can be calculated
at any age, being the average number of years which a person who
has reached that age can expect to live if the mortality rates for
people of that age and older ages neither increase nor decrease in
the future. In Britain, for example, the expectation of life of a forty
year old man in 1973 was 32.1 years, that of a seventy year old man
was 9.5 years, and the expectation of life for women was 37.5 years
and 12.6 years respectively. The death of a forty year old man,
therefore, can be said to represent a loss of 32.1 years and that of a
seventy year old man a loss of 9.5 years of expected life. Thus the
years of expected life which are lost for each person who dies and
for the whole community can be calculated. In Britain more than
half of the expected years are lost due to three diseases and nearly
three-quarters of years are lost due to only five types of disease.

Percentage of total less years of expected life

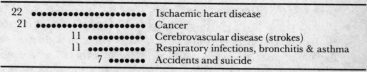

22 ●●●●●●●●●●●●●●●●●●●●●●●	Ischaemic heart disease
21 ●●●●●●●●●●●●●●●●●●●●●●	Cancer
11 ●●●●●●●●●●●	Cerebrovascular disease (strokes)
11 ●●●●●●●●●●●	Respiratory infections, bronchitis & asthma
7 ●●●●●●●	Accidents and suicide

Source: D.F.K. Black and J. D. Pole *British Journal of Social and Preventive Medicine*
(1975), Vol. 29.

Ischaemic heart disease

This is the commonest cause of death in most developed countries.
The basic pathological process is atherosclerosis, an accumulation

of fatty material in the walls of arteries. Many arteries are affected, particularly the cerebral vessels supplying the brain (see page 69), those supplying the muscles of the legs, causing pain in the calf muscles on walking called intermittent claudication, and those which supply the heart itself—the coronary arteries. Atherosclerosis narrows the coronary arteries reducing the rate of blood flow and causing oxygen starvation, ischaemia, of the muscular tissue of the heart. As the heart beats faster in exercise or in excitement it requires more blood and the effects of ischaemia are often first noticed at such times. The ischaemic muscle tissue which is starved of oxygen becomes painful and the pain, which is felt in the chest, neck, and left arm, is called angina. Chronic ischaemia can weaken the heart muscle resulting in heart failure, or an atherosclerotic artery can suddenly become completely blocked with the result that the heart muscle it supplies dies. Such an acute episode of ischaemia is called a heart attack and is sometimes fatal.

In 1976, the Royal College of Physicians of London and the British Cardiac Society issued a report on the 'Prevention of Coronary Heart Disease'. A number of recommendations to reduce the risk of ischaemic heart disease were made, the principal being:

- A reduction in the total dietary intake of fat and the substitution of foods rich in saturated fat such as fatty meat, egg yolks, butter, hard margerine, lard, and cream by poultry and fish as sources of protein, and polyunsaturated fats, such as sunflower oil, for cooking.
- The maintenance of an ideal body weight.
- A reduction in the amount of cigarette tobacco smoked, preferably by stopping completely.
- A graded increase in physical activity. The report recommends that the older person, the obese, and those with a history of cardiovascular disease should first consult their doctor but that most people do not need a medical examination before starting to exercise, provided they begin gently.

The report recorded the opinion that oral contraceptives constituted no more than a negligible risk for women under the age of forty but advised that they should be used with caution by women over forty or by women who were at risk in some other way, for example by being heavy cigarette smokers. It stated that doctors should pay particular attention to the blood pressure of those at risk and that 'while acute stress may occasionally precipitate a heart attack, it is difficult to prove that chronic stress contributes to the development of coronary heart disease', particularly emphasizing that 'initiative, diligence, leadership and hard work, especially in young people, should not be discouraged on the mistaken supposition that these qualities are indicators of future ischaemic heart disease'. The doctors who produced the report did not feel there was evidence to recommend dietary fibre as a means of prevention. Neither did research findings lead them to conclude that sugar or alcohol (except indirectly by causing obesity), coffee, salt, or hard water could be indited as causes of ischaemic heart disease.

The report has been widely accepted, but there are some differences of opinion. For example, some believe that not all these risk factors are of the same importance, maintaining that smoking and the dietary intake of saturated fats are the most significant and it is at them that preventive efforts should be directed. Others maintain that the initiation of programmes of prevention aimed at the whole community is inefficient and that prevention should be aimed at high risk groups, for example people with elevated levels of fat in their blood, and at people who will be strongly motivated to participate in the programme of prevention, such as relatives of people who have suffered a heart attack. However, these are minor points. There is general agreement not only that research has offered an opportunity for prevention but that a preventive approach is a necessity because further investment in hospital services will do little either to reduce the fatality of heart attacks or to cure the underlying disease of atherosclerosis.

It is encouraging that a decline in the mortality of man from ischaemic heart disease has been detected by an analysis of mortality statistics in the United States, Australia, and Great Britain. Only in the United States has a similar decline in the mortality of women been demonstrated. The decline, which started in 1968 in the United States and 1972 in Britain, cannot be attributed to any single preventive measure. British men have reduced their tobacco, sugar, and saturated fat consumption and they have taken more exercise in the last few years—all of which factors have probably played a part. The epidemic of ischaemic heart disease may have passed its zenith. Another recent encouraging trend is the prevention of disability following a heart attack. Doctors now appreciate that many of the measures previously employed in the treatment of a person who had had a heart attack, for example weeks of complete bed-rest followed by months off work, created a neurosis which was more disabling than the physical condition of the heart. A much more confident approach is now taken, often allowing the person out of bed within days of his attack, with his doctor encouraging him to consider an early return to normal work and life.

Cancer

The cells of most tissues are able to divide and reproduce exact copies of themselves. Even after the period of growth and development is finished this process takes place continuously in some tissues, for instance in the skin and bone marrow, while in others it occurs only following injury and cell death, for example bone cells can divide after a fracture. This process of normal cell division is under strict control. The new cells are situated only in the tissues in which they would be expected; for example, new bone cells do not spread into surrounding tissue, and the parent cells do not produce more new cells than is necessary to replace lost cells. In cancerous tissue this process is out of control. The cells which are produced are not only abnormal in both form and function but there is a tremendous over-production of cells at the site at which the cancer has started from a single cell, and the cancerous cells may spread throughout the body. Each cell or clump of cells which spreads gives rise to a new colony of cancer cells, called a metastasis, in whatever tissue it lands. Thus, lung cancer can spread to the bones and stomach cancer can spread to the liver by way of the bloodstream.

Cancers arise from single cells, the transition from normal cell function to the uncontrolled division and growth of cancer being the result of a number of factors. A causative factor, called a carcinogen, may be identifiable. For example, cigarette smoke certainly causes lung cancer but, as some smokers do not develop lung cancer and a proportion of those who develop cancer smoke less than some of those who do not, another factor or, more probably, other factors must also be at work.

Cancer has become an increasingly common cause of death in all developed countries. In part this can be explained by a decrease in deaths from other causes, notably infectious diseases, but more accurate recognition of the disease has also contributed to the increase in numbers of deaths registered as being due to cancer. After making allowance for such factors, however, it is evident that there has been a real increase in the numbers of people developing cancer. The most striking example is the increase of lung cancer in men and, some decades later, in women during the twentieth century as cigarette smoking became an increasingly prevalent habit. Such trends in time suggest that some cancers are caused by environmental factors and that there is, therefore, scope for prevention. Other evidence to support this theory is that there is no common cancer which is not rare in some part of the world. This could be due to genetic differences, but as it has been shown that some cancers become more common in a migrant group which moves from the country in which the cancer is uncommon to one in which it is common, it seems probable that environmental factors are responsible. Sir Richard Doll, the most eminent cancer epidemiologist, maintains that as many as ninety per cent of all cancers may be caused by environmental factors—not only pollutants, which are widely regarded with suspicion, but other factors which are not generally considered harmful. For example, melanoma, a type of skin cancer, noticed in several countries is possibly caused by the exposure of unpigmented skins to ultraviolet light from the sun.

Epidemiologists keep cancer deaths under review, looking for trends which might give clues. In this way the relationship between mesothelioma—cancer of the surface of the lung, which was rare in the 1950s but now causes about 200 deaths annually—and asbestos was established, but the cause, or causes, of many cancers remains unknown. Cancer of the stomach, for example, which killed 6,925 men and 4,944 women in England and Wales during 1976, varies widely from one part of the world to another and is decreasing quite quickly in Britain; but the reason for the decrease, which would illuminate the cause of stomach cancer, has not yet been determined. In spite of the fact that the causes of many cancers are unknown, a number of opportunities exist for the primary prevention of cancer.

Common cancers in which preventable factors have been identified or are under suspicion, England and Wales 1976

	Men		Women		Causal factors
	Annual number of deaths	Percentage of all cancer deaths	Annual number of deaths	Percentage of all cancer deaths	
Trachea, bronchus, and lung	26,579	42.8	6,947	11.8	Cigarette smoking is responsible for over 90 per cent of lung cancer. Industrial exposure to asbestos, nickel, and chrome, can also cause cancer.
Colon	4,461	7.2	6,335	10.8	Not known: possibly a diet which contains a high amount of meat and low amount of cereal fibre.
Rectum	3,337	5.4	2,920	4.9	Not known: possibly the same factors implicated in cancer of the colon.
Bladder	2,951	4.8	1,291	2.2	Smoking and certain aniline dyes in industry (see p. 71).
Oesophagus	1,936	3.1	1,516	2.6	Smoking and alcohol
Mouth and throat	996	1.6	638	1.0	Smoking and alcohol
Melanoma	324	0.5	457	0.8	Ultraviolet light

					Comment
Breast	68	–	11,763	20	Those women who have their first pregnancy under the age of 20 have a lower risk than those who have first pregnancy over the age of 30 but the causal factor is not known.
Cervix of the uterus (neck of the womb)	–	–	2,206	3.7	This is more common in women who started sexual intercourse earlier and the risk increases as the number of sexual partners increases, but the causal mechanism is not known. (It is possible that it is infection with herpes virus, which also causes cold sores round the mouth. If this were so, cancer of the cervix could be considered a complication of a veneral disease.)
Body of the uterus	–	–	1,501	2.6	Hormone replacement therapy given for menopausal symptoms substantially increases the risk.
Total	62,023	100	58,758	100	

Primary prevention of some cancers can be achieved comparatively easily. It is relatively simple to persuade some doctors not to prescribe hormones indiscriminately to women with minor symptoms, and it is possible, although it can be expensive and difficult, to protect industrial workers from harmful chemicals. It is much more difficult, however, to influence smoking habits—the main opportunity for primary prevention—or to affect the sexual habits of young people.

Secondary prevention—the attempt to detect cancer at an earlier, presymptomatic stage—has also been attempted. The most successful programme of secondary prevention is that of screening all the women in a population for evidence of the early stages of cancer of the cervix (the neck of the womb). Cells are scraped from the surface of the cervix and examined for evidence of early cancer, a procedure known as cervical cytology. If cancer is detected at an early stage before it has invaded the underlying tissue, a small section of the cervix is removed. This extirpates the cancer but does not interfere with the woman's ability to bear children. Although there were some doubts about the effectiveness of this approach in the early stages of the screening programme, there is now firm evidence that cancer of the cervix is preventable by cervical screening. The main drawback is that those who are most at risk, for example women past child-bearing age, use the service less than younger women who are less at risk. To reduce the number of cases of cancer further research is needed to ascertain the reasons why some women do not accept the opportunity of the cervical smear test which is free, painless, and takes only a few minutes. The reasons may be practical, such as difficulty in reaching the clinic, or psychological, such as a belief that all cancer is hopeless and incurable and that the early detection of cancer of the cervix is useless (see page 148).

Because cancer of the breast is often advanced when the woman affected first attends the doctor and because it can be detected at an early stage, screening for breast cancer may be beneficial, but no decision has yet been reached on whether or not it should be introduced as a national service (see page 140).

Secondary prevention by screening may be feasible if the risk is high in a definable population. Although it would be impractical to study the urine of every cigarette smoker to see if it contained cancerous cells (an early sign of bladder cancer which develops before there is pain or bleeding), cytological screening of those people who are exposed to certain aniline chemicals in the manufacture of dyes, rubber antioxidants, and elastomers in the plastics industry is worthwhile because the risk of bladder cancer is high in that group of people. Similarly, although it is considered inappropriate in the U. K. to X-ray the stomach of every person for evidence of early stomach cancer, in Japan, where stomach cancer is six times more common, being responsible for 44 per cent of all male cancer deaths and 36 per cent of all female cancer deaths, such a screening programme is relevant and has been instituted, although it must be said that its value has not yet been clearly demonstrated. Similarly, in parts of China where cancer of the oesophagus is common a screening programme has been instituted, but it would not be started in Britain where that type of cancer is rare.

There are hopeful signs. A decline in the number of people affected by stomach cancer has been reported from a number of countries, although the reason for this decline is as mysterious as the cause of the cancer. Even more encouraging is the fact that in England and Wales in 1975 the number of men dying of lung cancer decreased for the first time in fifty years, reflecting the decrease in cigarette smoking. Unfortunately the number of women affected showed yet another increase, continuing a remorseless upward trend and reflecting the increasing tobacco consumption of women in previous decades. Even within the limits of our present state of knowledge there are many opportunities for preventing cancer, and the main one is the prevention of cigarette smoking (see page 160).

Cerebrovascular disease

Because nerve cells are unable to divide and replace those which die, brain damage is irreparable and, because the brain is such an important organ, it is often fatal. The commonest cause of brain damage is cerebrovascular disease which interferes with the blood supply to the brain. The flow of blood containing dissolved oxygen may be interrupted by either a blood clot in an artery or the rupture of an artery, with haemorrhage of blood into the brain substance. A sudden interruption of the blood supply is called a cerebrovascular accident—a stroke. A stroke is not necessarily fatal. Many people survive, usually with some residual disability, but death frequently results. Many factors can predispose to a cerebrovascular accident but two are common—atherosclerosis (see page 63), which damages and weakens the arterial walls, and high blood pressure. The prevention of atherosclerosis in the cerebral blood vessels is possible and the measures suggested in the report of the Royal College of Physicians and the British Cardiac Society to prevent atherosclerosis in the arteries of the heart (see page 64) are also important in the prevention of atherosclerosis in the blood vessels supplying the brain, but established atherosclerosis, for instance in a man aged fifty, is probably impossible to reverse. High blood pressure, on the other hand can be reversed.

One of the triumphs of pharmacology has been the development of effective drugs to lower blood pressure, but before high blood pressure can be treated it has to be diagnosed and this is not always easy. Blood pressure is simple to measure with a sphygmomanometer but the interpretation of the measurement can present problems. Blood pressure is as much a physical characteristic as height. In any population in which blood pressure is measured there will be a range of values, just as there is a range of heights. The most common blood pressure is the average, but the majority of people have a pressure which is not average: some are normally lower than average, others are normally higher. The higher the blood pressure the greater the risk of a stroke, but there is no value of blood pressure at which normal blood pressure ends and high blood pressure begins. 'High blood pressure' is not a distinct physical condition as is infection by malarial parasites or a broken bone. The 'disease' is distinguished from the 'normal' state by medical convention at a value above which doctors believe that the benefits of treatment outweigh the side-effects, for not only do the drugs used to lower blood pressure have other physical effects but psychological problems can develop from being told that one has high blood pressure and must take treatment for the rest of one's life.

At levels of blood pressure very much higher than the average doctors are unanimous in agreeing that treatment is necessary. At lower levels, which are nearer the average, there is, however, uncertainty about the benefits of treatment and the Medical

Research Council (M.R.C.) is currently organizing a clinical trial of the treatment of moderately above average blood pressure. Even if this trial shows a statistically clear-cut benefit between the group in which people are treated compared with the group in which they are not, the individual doctor detecting that a person has blood pressure moderately above average will still have a difficult decision to make. The significance of an individual's blood pressure depends on a number of factors, of which the conclusion drawn from the results of treatment given to a group of people with the same blood pressure in a research project, such as the M.R.C. trial, is only one. The doctor has also to consider the person's age, weight, whether he has diabetes or smokes, whether he has a relative who had a stroke, and a number of other factors. The decision will always require clinical judgement.

There is scope for prevention even though this question is unresolved. There are people who would definitely benefit from treatment, having a blood pressure very much above average which has never been detected because very elevated blood pressure does not always make its presence known by causing symptoms. Attempts to measure the blood pressure of everyone in a defined population, for example a city, to find those people with undetected high blood pressure has been suggested, but the approach adopted so far is to encourage doctors to take the opportunity to measure the blood pressure whenever anyone consults, whatever the person's reason for consultation. It is particularly important to check the blood pressure when a woman attends a family planning clinic because oral contraceptives can increase blood pressure.

In 1978 clinical research suggested that, although the anti-coagulant drugs usually used in medicine did not prevent thrombosis in the arteries of the brain, aspirin, which affects the blood's clotting properties in addition to its analgesic function, might prevent strokes in those people in whom the early signs of stroke had been detected. This is an exciting finding which may lead to stroke prevention although it should not be forgotten that a very important aspect of prevention takes place after the stroke has occurred. Careful medical and nursing care, skilled occupational and speech therapy, physiotherapy, and sensitive social work can prevent disability and handicap by minimizing the secondary effects of the brain damage (see page 86).

Respiratory infections, bronchitis, and asthma

Antibiotics now prevent many deaths from pneumonia in young people but pneumonia is still recorded as a common cause of death in old people. To some extent this is misleading because the lung infection which terminates the life of an old person is often secondary to the accumulation of fluid in the lungs as a result of heart failure, so that respiratory infection is a secondary cause of death. Antibiotics have prevented many other problems, for example by preventing many mild cases of tonsillitis becoming severe. The number of tonsillectomy operations has decreased markedly in the last two decades although this is also due to a change in medical fashion: doctors no longer remove tonsils as readily as they did formerly. The treatment of tonsillitis with antibiotics has contributed to the prevention of rheumatic fever. This is a sequel to infection of the tonsils by certain types of streptococcal bacteria which can stimulate the body to produce antibodies (see page 10) against its own heart tissue. It is also possible that there has been a natural decline in the virulence of such streptococci (see page 5). These factors have not only reduced mortality from acute rheumatic fever but they have also reduced the number of people with chronic rheumatic heart disease which was a common cause of death and disability in people who survived the acute stage of rheumatic fever.

The suffix '-itis', meaning inflammation, usually implies infection, as in tonsillitis, which is bacterial inflammation of the tonsils. Bronchitis is thus inflammation of the bronchial tubes. Acute bronchitis is usually bacterial in origin, chronic bronchitis is not. Although the airways become infected more easily because of chronic bronchitis, the illness does not develop as a result of infection. The pathology of chronic bronchitis is not uniform. The main feature may be an excessive production of mucus which predisposes to infection by bacteria which would not infect someone with normal mucus production. Alternatively it may be a narrowing of the air passages resulting in wheezing, sometimes called asthmatic bronchitis, or, the third variant, lung tissue may be lost resulting in emphysema, larger than normal air spaces in the lung. In most people with bronchitis all three features are present but the pattern varies from one patient to another.

Although bronchitis causes about 30,000 deaths every year, this is only one aspect of the disease. One million people have chronic bronchitis and one-tenth of the days of work lost are classified as being due to bronchitis. In 1974 the treatment of bronchitis cost the National Health Service £100 million, the cost of lost production was probably in the region of £250 million, and £56 million of social security payments were paid out because of bronchitis.

There are three main causes of chronic bronchitis—air pollution, dusty working conditions, and cigarette smoking. Industrial Britain was black with the smoke of factory and domestic fires and one of the consequences of the industrial revolution was the rise of bronchitis. In some cities it became so familiar that a productive cough came to be regarded as a normal concomitant of ageing, but the Clean Air Acts of 1956 and 1968, consolidated by the Control of Pollution Act 1974, dramatically reduced the levels of air pollution. Between 1952 and 1965 smoke emission fell from 2.39 million metric tons per annum to 0.39 million metric tons. From 1969 to 1975 the amount of particulate matter in the air fell by about half and the amount of sulphur dioxide decreased by about one-third. This cleaning of the air will have a long-term pay-off in addition to the benefits already obtained because one of the effects of air pollution is to initiate bronchitic changes in the lungs of children.

There is a marked difference in the frequency with which bronchitis affects workers in different occupations. The standardized mortality ratio of chronic bronchitis allows comparison with the bronchitis mortality rate of the total population, making allowance for any differences between the age range of the defined group and the age range of the total population. It is a form of percentage, the standardized mortality ratio (S.M.R.) for the whole population is 100 but it is over 200 for miners, and over 150 for dockers, engineering labourers, and furnacemen. It is, however, less than 50 for mine managers and engineering managers. Bronchitis which is caused by dust encountered at work should not be confused with pneumoconiosis, the deposition of dust in the lungs, which is a separate condition although it often co-exists with bronchitis. By the introduction of techniques such as the wetting of stone which is being cut, and the substitution of men with machines for certain tasks, the exposure of workers to dust has decreased but will continue to be an occupational health hazard (see page 105).

Cigarette smoking is now the main cause of bronchitis in Britain affecting not only the smoker but his children, who develop respiratory problems more frequently than the children of non-smokers. Cigarette smoke now causes more bronchitis than all the other causes added together and the prevention of bronchitis depends upon the reduction of cigarette smoking (see page 160).

Asthma is a tendency for the airways to narrow suddenly. Some people are genetically predisposed to react abnormally to certain normal substances, a type of response known as an allergic reaction. The usual material which stimulates this allergic reaction and causes asthma is protein from the house dust mite, which is a very common and usually harmless creature. Psychological stress can increase the severity of this allergic reaction and infection by viruses or bacteria can aggravate asthma. Primary prevention is only successful when there is an allergic substance which can be easily avoided or removed from the environment, such as horse dander or feathers, which is not the case with the ubiquitous house dust mite. The amount of disability caused by asthma has been reduced as its treatment has improved in the last thirty years due to the introduction of drugs which can relieve the spasm of the airways, especially bronchodilator aerosols, and antibiotics which effectively treat the infections that so often complicate the disease. However, the mortality from asthma has not decreased significantly this century, although there is evidence that deaths can be prevented if acute attacks are recognized and referred for hospital treatment at an early stage.

The steady decline in tuberculosis has already been discussed but the disease is by no means extinct. New sources of infection are brought into Britain by immigrants and a pool of infection survives among homeless alcoholics who are not only particularly susceptible to infection but are difficult to treat as their mobile and unstable lifestyle prevents the careful supervision of treatment which is required to cure the disease. However, tuberculosis is now a minor problem in comparison with the respiratory diseases which are known to be caused by cigarette smoking and, for many people, a lesser worry than the possibility that new types of air pollution, although they are no longer in the obvious form of black smoke and fog, may contain chemicals which damage the respiratory system.

Accidents and suicide

The word accident implies unpredictability—but accidents usually have identifiable causes and are often preventable. They are either the unconsidered consequences of actions or they are consequences which were foreseen but which were considered so improbable that no steps were taken to prevent them. For example, a driver may skid on a wet road because he had not considered the effect of rain on the road surface, or he may skid because he assumed that the amount of alcohol he had consumed would not impair his driving skill on wet roads.

Accidents on the road

Each year in Britain 100,000 people are admitted to hospital having been injured on the road—80,000 people are seriously injured, and more than 6,600 die. Although these figures seem shockingly high there has been a great improvement in road safety in the last twenty years. Since 1961 the number of vehicles licensed in Great Britain and the total mileage travelled has almost doubled, yet the number of people killed and injured has not increased, but in fact decreased by a small amount.

	1961	1976
Licensed vehicles	10.0 million	17.8 million
Index of vehicle mileage (1966 = 100 per cent)	71 per cent	145 per cent
People killed	6,900	6,600
People seriously injured	85,000	80,800
People slightly injured	258,000	254,000

Source: *Social Trends* (H.M.S.O., 1977).

The preventive measures responsible have been of many different types. The educational efforts of the police, road safety officers, and driving instructors; safer car design; an increasingly comprehensive and strict code of legislation governing the condition of cars on the road; an improvement in the quality of the road network and street lighting; and the legislation which made the wearing of crash helmets compulsory, have all had their influence. With so many identifiable factors to explain this improvement it is difficult to assess whether or not the behaviour of road users— drivers, cyclists, and pedestrians—has improved, but it is the conduct of road users, particularly their consideration for the safety of, and courtesy towards, other road users, which is as important as their skills, the condition of the roads, or their vehicles in determining whether or not they cause accidents. Britain compares well with other developed countries yet there is still considerable scope for prevention. The relative risk, and therefore the scope for prevention, is greatest for cyclists and riders of motor cycles.

Type of vehicle	Number of people killed or seriously injured per 100 million vehicle kilometres in 1976
Pedal cyclists	126,000
Motor cyclists	308,000
Drivers of cars and taxis	10,000
Drivers of goods vehicles	6,000
Drivers of public service vehicles	4,000

Source: *Social Trends* (H.M.S.O., 1977).

Accidents are more common in men than in women and in younger drivers and motor cyclists, and those at greatest relative risk are young men on motor bikes. Various preventative measures have been discussed, such as the introduction of tighter restrictions on the use of bikes of higher cubic capacity, but the challenge to prevention is formidable because the basic problem is the risk-taking behaviour of young men, which is a feature of many societies (see page 148). It is probable, however, that the driving test is too easy and that an investment of more public money in compulsory education for all motor bike riders, combined with a more stringent examination of their skill in difficult conditions, would reduce this very high rate. The police and county councils are trying to increase the amount of education given to young motor cyclists, but their efforts have been limited by public expenditure cuts. The R.A.C.– A.C.U. (Auto Cyclists Union) national training scheme is limited by the lack of suitable training grounds, and S.T.E.P. (Schools Transport Educational Programme) is limited by a shortage of trained instructors. Local authority road safety training officers working in the Surveyor's department suffered in the series of public expenditure cuts which followed the OPEC increase in oil prices in 1973—cuts which particularly affected the highways services, the main responsibility of the County Surveyor. The motor bike industry has shown a welcome willingness to fund S.T.E.P. projects, but the numbers of experienced road safety training officers and police officers able to train motorcyclists and to educate other people to perform the training, such as teachers, is too few in the face of the increasing numbers of young motor cyclists.

Although drivers and passengers of cars are at much less risk, there are so many more cars than motor bikes on the road that more than twice as many people are killed or seriously injured in cars than on bikes.

Persons killed or seriously injured by class of road users, Great Britain 1976

Pedestrians		20,500
Pedal cyclists		4,900
Two wheeled motor vehicle	riders	17,900
	passengers	1,900
Four wheeled motor vehicle	drivers	22,100
	passengers	18,400

Source: *Social Trends* (H.M.S.O, 1977).

The government's Transport and Road Research Laboratory has high-lighted many possible means of reducing the toll, from which two major measures stand out—the prevention of drinking and driving and the introduction of legislation to make the wearing of seat belts compulsory.

In 1968, legislation was introduced which made it compulsory for seat belts to be fitted on new motor cars but a survey in 1974 found that no more than 27 per cent of drivers wore seat belts, the proportion being 39 per cent on motorway journeys. By 1978, after a period in which a considerable amount of money had been spent on advertisements, the Secretary of State for Transport stated in the Commons that the proportion had increased to only 31 per cent. If all drivers wore seat belts the estimated annual saving would be 1,000 lives and 12,000 serious injuries to people of all ages. During 1974, 2,260 children under 15 years were killed or seriously injured in cars, yet a survey in the same year found that only 13 per cent of children were restrained while travelling. Although there is evidence to suggest that as many as 85 per cent of deaths and 70 per cent of the serious injuries of children could be prevented if restraints were worn, this situation has been allowed to continue with very little comment by the public or in the press. In March 1978 another advertising campaign, costing £700,000, was launched to encourage people to wear seat belts but many people believe that the problem should be tackled by legislation not education.

Legislation to make the wearing of seat belts compulsory has been vigorously opposed. The necessary proposals have entered both Houses of Parliament but have not reached the statute book. Although there is little dispute that the measure would save lives, opposition has been on ethical grounds. The opponents of legislation claim that such a matter as an individual's decision whether or not to wear a seat belt should be determined not by law but by the individual concerned (see page 157).

The Road Traffic Act of 1967 introduced the breathalyser and its preventive effect was dramatic. In 1966 almost 40 per cent of drivers aged between 20 and 40 killed on the road had had blood alcohol levels greater than 80 mgm per 100 ml. In the year after the introduction of the breath test the proportion for this age group was only 20 per cent. It is estimated that 1,000 lives were saved in the first year after the Act became law and 4,000 lives and 200,000 casualties were prevented in subsequent years, but the preventive effect soon diminished. By 1974, 35 per cent of drivers killed in this age group had levels above the legal limit and by 1977 the proportion had risen to a level which was higher than before the 1967 Act. In 1974, aware of the escalating problem, the Department of the Environment convened a Committee to investigate Drinking and Driving. The Blennerhassett Committee, so called after its chairman, recommended that drinking and driving should be considered in the wider context of all the problems of alcohol abuse, and that the powers of the police should be extended, but little came of their recommendations. Although large sums of money have been spent exhorting drivers not to drink and drive, £500,000 in 1977, the effectiveness of this approach remains unproven. This is one area of prevention in which greater government action appears to be essential, although the steps which it could take are not so obvious as in the seat belt issue. Stopping and breathalysing motorists at random, instead of the present approach of breath testing only those who are committing a road traffic offence or are giving rise to suspicion, has been suggested, and has been introduced in France, but it is not considered that such a move would be effective in Britain. Those who drink and drive with serious consequences are not just individuals who have had three drinks rather than two. They are usually people who are heavy drinkers and they not infrequently have other problems associated with chronic excessive consumption of alcohol: their driving problems have to be considered in the spectrum of the other problems of alcohol abuse (see page 165).

Seat belts and the drinking driver are only two issues among many which have to be considered. Road deaths in France, for example, have decreased by 20 per cent in spite of a 30 per cent increase in traffic, not only because of the mandatory use of seat belts but because of the lower speed limits. In Britain there was a 14 per cent decrease in the number of people killed or seriously injured on the road between 1973 and 1975. In spite of the fact that this was almost certainly due in part to the lower speed limits imposed during that period for energy conservation the Secretary of State for Transport announced on 6 April 1977 that the limits were to be raised to their previous levels thus discarding a preventive measure which had been fortuitously implemented. It is important to emphasize that no matter what external constraints are applied the crucial factor is internal: the drivers' attitudes. The safe driver is one who considers not only his own safety but that of other people.

More than 25,000 pedestrians and cyclists are killed or severely injured every year. The two groups most at risk are elderly people and children. More than 80 per cent of the children injured or killed are hit while crossing a road, one-quarter of them in the road in which they live. Although the government spent £880,000 in the winter of 1976 to increase their safety consciousness, the problem probably requires more direct action. Britain has the worst child pedestrian casualty rate in western Europe.

There is no statutory test for children who wish to ride bicycles, but the National Cycling Proficiency Scheme, promoted by the Cyclists Touring Club, the British Cycling Federation, and the Royal Society for the Prevention of Accidents (RoSPA), instructs and tests children in bicycle control and road safety. In 1975, 255,000 children passed this test, but much more could be done if police road safety officers and others who teach children and young pedestrians were given more financial resources.

Accidents at work (see page 106)

Accidents at home and at play

In the United Kingdom more than 6,500 people die as a result of accidents at home and at play. The groups most at risk are children and elderly people.

In England and Wales in 1973, 101 children died as a result of a fall; 143 died as a result of burns; 192 choked to death; 84 suffocated; 198 drowned; 34 were poisoned; and 102 died as a result of purposefully inflicted injury. Younger children, those under 5 years of age, are particularly at risk, but as children grow older a decreasing proportion die at home which becomes relatively less dangerous than road traffic. Not only fatalities should be considered. 142,000 children were admitted to hospitals in England and Wales as a result of accidents in 1974 and no estimate can be made of the anguish and suffering of parents and children.

Sometimes a cause can be clearly identified and it is to be hoped that the home accident surveillance programme, instituted in 1977 by the Consumer Safety Unit of the Department of Prices and Consumer Protection, will reveal more environmental factors which can be modified. If it can, prevention may be possible. The use of childproof containers for prescribed drugs and medicines, for instance, should reduce not only the mortality from poisoning but the number of hospital admissions—16,000 in 1972—but it has been found that the accident often results not only from a child's physical environment but from his social environment. Accidents can occur to the children of the most careful and caring parents but children whose parents care less are more at risk and this predisposing factor is not one easily modified by preventive medicine.

Death rates from accidents in the home, 1974

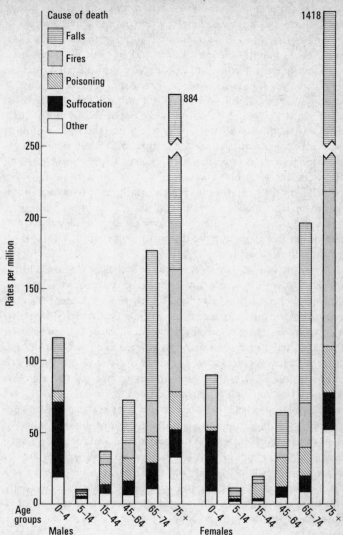

¹ Includes accidents caused by explosive material, fireworks, blasting material, explosive gases, hot substances, corrosive liquid, electric shocks, etc.
Source: *Mortality Statistics: accidents and violence*, Office of Population Censuses and Surveys (H.M.S.O., 1974)

Even specially designed playgrounds have their danger. The Research Institute for Consumer Affairs has estimated that about 150,000 children require treatment by a doctor or hospital admission each year because of injuries sustained in playgrounds. Fair Play for Children, a group specially interested in play facilities, also collected evidence on the dangers of play equipment which it presented to the Department of the Environment. As a result of these and similar findings, new British Standards for Permanently Installed Outdoor Play Equipment were produced by the British Standards Institution and these should reduce the risk, although safe equipment is no substitute for trained play leaders and play-ground supervisors. A study by the Office of Population Censuses and Surveys on the mortality of children in England and Wales between 1970 and 1972 found that the mortality rate from accidents and violence was nearly five times as high for the children of unskilled parents than for the children of professional parents, the greatest difference being for deaths as a result of fires, followed by deaths of child pedestrians.

Accidents in old age have both medical and environmental causes. For example, some fires could be prevented if elderly people were helped to replace paraffin heaters with gas fires or if they were encouraged to use local authority maturity loans to replace dangerous electric wiring, and some falls could be prevented if house lighting was improved and rails were fixed on both sides of the stairway. However, because the sense of balance is impaired in some elderly people, they may trip and fall no matter how safe their environment. Nevertheless, careful attention to the visual and medical problems of old people can prevent some accidents by improving an elderly person's ability to maintain her sense of balance, see dangers, take steps to avoid them, and recover balance before she falls if she should trip. The common consequence of a fall is a fractured femur, which usually requires operative repair, and it is the effects of blood loss and the pneumonia, which can occur easily in immobilized old people, that are the usual causes of death rather than the direct result of the accident.

Suicide

Suicide is common in every developed country. It is more common in men than in women and the death rate in both sexes increases with age, becoming higher the older the age group considered. The suicide rate of men is lower than it has been at any time this century but in women the rate is one-third higher than it was in 1901. Since 1963 mortality from suicide has decreased, but this decrease has been more marked in the old age groups, the death rate having increased in men aged between 15 and 25.

The suicide rates in different periods are not exactly comparable because the certification of suicide as the cause of death was, and is, influenced by many factors. Before 1961 attempted suicide was a criminal offence so it was not always reported. Since then, although suicide is no longer a criminal offence, it still has a social stigma and is therefore sometimes concealed to spare relatives' feelings. In spite of these qualifications the decrease appears to be real. It can be explained neither by a change in the classification of cause of death nor by the more effective treatment which is now given, that is the decrease in the death rate cannot be completely explained by the survival of cases who would have previously died.

The introduction of North Sea gas has been suggested as a cause of the decline and deaths from gas poisoning have indeed fallen sharply, but it is probable that a person determined to commit suicide would use an alternative method if he knew that poisoning by gas was no longer effective. More likely reasons are the activities of the Samaritans—the number of people saying that they are considering suicide who phone the Samaritans increased five-fold between 1964 and 1970—and the more effective medical and social treatment of depression. These are identifiable factors but there are probably many others which are less easy to identify. Suicide rates fluctuate in all societies, usually rising in time of economic uncertainty and falling in time of war when the bonds of society are strengthened and individuals have a sense of belonging and purpose. Suicide has fascinated sociologists since Durkheim wrote his classic study of the phenomenon, but the sociological explanation of suicide, and any possibilities for prevention which such an explanation might offer, is still a matter of debate.

Although the number of deaths from suicide is decreasing, the number of people who attempt suicide is increasing very rapidly. People who attempt suicide can be classified in two groups. There are those whose intent is serious who have usually considered the action over a period of time before making the final decision and who try to commit suicide in a way which they are confident will be effective. The probability of death is high in this group. The other group consists of people who do not attempt suicide as a result of prolonged deliberation but as an impulsive action. The action is often publicized, either before or after the event, in a way which ensures that help will be called and the method chosen is frequently of a nature which is known, consciously or unconsciously, to be unlikely to have a fatal outcome, for example the consumption of ten aspirins. The motive of people in this group, whose intent to kill themselves is not serious, is not so much an act of self-punishment as one which has the intention, conscious or unconscious, of influencing other people by making them feel guilty or sympathetic. The probability of a fatal outcome is much lower in this group and it is this type of suicide, sometimes called para-suicide, which accounts for the increase in the number of cases of attempted suicide. Para-suicide is more common in younger age groups, especially among young women, and because the action is so frequently impulsive, prevention is very difficult.

Prevention of disability

Physical disability

It is common to talk about 'the disabled' or 'disabled people' as though disability was a distinct condition of people in a separate class in society, but disability is relative. Every individual, no matter how strong or skilled he may be, is less able than someone else in some sphere of physical or mental activity, but a person is usually considered to be 'disabled' when disease significantly impairs his ability in comparison not only with his abilities before disease affected him, but also with what is reasonable for someone of his age to expect to be able to do. He can be said to be 'handicapped' if the disability interferes with his ability to look after himself, work, or enjoy leisure pursuits in a manner which would normally be expected by someone of his age.

Handicap is also relative. It not only depends upon the degree of disability but on the social and physical environment in which the person with impaired function lives. For example, a person in a wheelchair who is able to study at a university department because it has been designed without any steps at the entrances and with lifts to all floors, is not handicapped in his education, but he would have been handicapped if the architects had designed the campus of his choice on many different levels for aesthetic effects and had omitted lifts from the building. Similarly a woman who has severe arthritis in the knees and hips but who is able to go to the toilet independently because it is on the ground floor is not handicapped in this aspect of her life, although she would be handicapped if she happened to live in a house in which the toilet was in the back garden or at the top of a flight of stairs she could not climb. It is useful and important to distinguish between disability and handicap because the environmental factors which cause handicap are often easier to prevent than the diseases which cause disability.

The great majority of people who are handicapped by physical

	Men	Women	Most common cause
Very severely handicapped	45,000	113,000	One-half of the men and one-third of the women in this category were disabled by diseases of the central nervous system of which the most common by far was cerebro-vascular disease (see page 71).
Severely handicapped	145,000	367,000	Arthritis was the cause of disability of 40 per cent of this group.

Source: *Handicapped and Impaired in Great Britain*, Office of Population Censuses and Surveys (H.M.S.O., 1971).

disability live at home supported by family, friends, volunteers, neighbours, and the community health and social services, with only occasional stays in hospital. The extent of disability in the community was not realized until the Office of Population Census and Survey's *Handicapped and Impaired in Great Britain* investigation was conducted by Amelia Harris in the winter of 1968. The survey tried to determine the number of people who were handicapped, that is the criteria used were functional not medical. People were asked if they could dress, undress, wash, bathe, and go to the toilet independently, or whether they required assistance with any or all of these functions. The survey also asked about housing and employment and ascertained how many people were too immobilized by their disability to enjoy leisure activities reasonable for people of their age. 670,000 people were found to be either severely or very severely handicapped, although still living at home. Those who were very severely handicapped required assistance with the basic activities of life regularly throughout the day and, for some people, throughout the night also. Those classified as severely disabled required less help but were still unable to manage at home independently.

In people over the age of 65, arthritis, stroke, Parkinson's disease, blindness, and heart disease are the most common causes of disability, and many very elderly people are simultaneously affected by more than one of these diseases. In the age group 50-64 years, arthritis and stroke are also common causes of disability but other diseases of the nervous system, particularly paraplegia, that is paralysis from the waist down due to damage to the spinal cord, and multiple sclerosis, are relatively more common than in older people. Chronic bronchitis and heart disease are also frequent causes of disability, especially in men. In people aged under 50 but over 16 years stroke is an uncommon cause of physical disability but arthritis, multiple sclerosis, and paraplegia are the common causes of severe physical disability, together with the effects of accidents and congenital handicap because some children who have been severely handicapped from birth survive to become handicapped adults. Arthritis is the commonest cause of physical disability in people of working age.

Percentage of disability of people aged 15–65

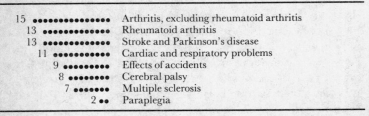

15 ●●●●●●●●●●●●●●●	Arthritis, excluding rheumatoid arthritis
13 ●●●●●●●●●●●●●	Rheumatoid arthritis
13 ●●●●●●●●●●●●●	Stroke and Parkinson's disease
11 ●●●●●●●●●●●	Cardiac and respiratory problems
9 ●●●●●●●●●	Effects of accidents
8 ●●●●●●●●	Cerebral palsy
7 ●●●●●●●	Multiple sclerosis
2 ●●	Paraplegia

Source: *Physical Impairment and Social Handicap* (Office of Health Economics, 1977), p. 10.

Younger people suffer from rheumatoid arthritis, which affects women about four times as frequently as men. A great deal has been discovered about the mechanism by which the joints are damaged. The immune system which normally attacks invading viruses and bacteria attacks the joints instead, causing inflammation and destruction, but the cause of rheumatoid arthritis is still unknown. In spite of the fact that the disease cannot be prevented, the disability which results from damaged joints can be greatly reduced by good medical care. Doctors now have at their disposal drugs which can control the inflammatory process and artificial joints which can be used to replace those which have been severely damaged by the immune system's destructive activity. The correct use of these new therapeutic opportunities, together with skilled occupational and physiotherapy, can prevent disability and pain. However, the specialist rheumatology services necessary to make the best use of these medical advances are very unequally distributed between the different regions of Britain. In some parts of the country it is comparatively easy for G.P.s to refer patients to see a consultant rheumatologist; in other parts the waiting list is very long. In some areas there are no consultant rheumatologists. The affected person's access to this form of preventive medicine depends, however, not only on the availability of specialist services but on her G.P.'s willingness to refer her for an expert opinion, and this is determined by his knowledge of, and interest in, rheumatoid arthritis. This varies from one G.P. to another, but is being improved due to better training of general practitioners.

In older people the most common type of joint disease is osteo-arthritis, which is perhaps inappropriately called arthritis because the disease process is not so much an inflammatory, as the suffix '-itis' suggests, as a degenerative process. It is the wearing away of the smooth cartilage which covers the end of the bone at the joint surface. The cartilage firstly wears thin and then wears away completely exposing bone which is not only rougher than cartilage but is sensitive to pain, which cartilage is not. The result is stiffness, due to the increased friction, and pain. Osteoarthritis affects almost everyone as they age but some people are very much more affected than others. Obesity puts an increased load on the weight bearing joints of spine, hips, knees, and feet which are the joints most commonly affected by osteoarthritis, and is the main preventable factor (see page 107). But as many thin people are also affected there must be other causal factors, some of them probably genetic, which determine the rate at which cartilage wears out. Although there are no drugs which can arrest the degeneration of the joint cartilage, as there are drugs to control the inflammatory rheumatoid process, medical treatment is also preventive because the control of pain by careful drug therapy allows the affected individual to remain mobile, and this prevents joint stiffness, as can physiotherapy. In severe cases surgical replacement of the hip joint by the artificial hip, the hip prosthesis, developed by Sir John Charnley, prevents disability.

Multiple sclerosis is a disease of nervous tissue which can attack any part of the central nervous system so that the symptoms vary very much from one person to another. Weakness, paralysis, tremor, uncoordinated movements, or blindness may occur and all are disabling. The signs and symptoms of the disease vary not only from one person to another but change from time to time in the same person because the symptoms of multiple sclerosis fluctuate in severity. As the cause is unknown prevention is impossible at present but there are hopeful findings from recent research. It is now thought that multiple sclerosis may be a response to a viral infection, perhaps an uncommon reaction to a very common virus which causes only minor symptons in the great majority of people but which causes multiple sclerosis in a minority whose response to infection is abnormal. If the cause could be found prevention might be possible. Parkinson's disease affects those parts of the brain which control and co-ordinate movement. Muscles become tense, and movements are slow and complicated by tremor. In some people the disease is caused by atherosclerosis of the arteries leading to these co-ordinating centres in the brain and is therefore preventable if atherosclerosis is prevented (see page 77) but in the majority of cases no cause can be identified, so prevention is impossible. The most common preventable cause of paraplegic paralysis is injury on the road but no specific type of accident is particularly associated with fracture of the spine and severance of the spinal cord so the prevention of paraplegia depends upon the prevention of all types of accident rather than on the introduction of any specific measure (see page 77). Although these diseases of nervous tissue offer little scope for prevention, specialist and skilled medical treatment can minimize disability. The appropriate use of drugs in the management of people with multiple sclerosis and Parkinson's disease, the prevention of bladder infection and skin ulceration in people who are paraplegic, and skilled physiotherapy are important preventive measures, but primary prevention is impossible until epidemiologists, virologists, biochemists, and other research workers discover the primary causes of these disabling diseases.

Skilled treatment may reduce disability to a level at which the individual, though disabled, is independently able to care for himself, to work, or to get about from place to place. Very disabled people, however, are often handicapped in these basic activities and occupational therapists are trained to prevent such handicaps. The first approach of the therapist is to try to teach the disabled person a new way of performing the task which disability has made impossible, for example a new method of putting on a jacket. If this fails she may be able to provide an aid, for example a lever which can enable someone with a weak handgrip to turn taps on and off. Sometimes neither teaching new skills nor the provision of aids are sufficient and it is often necessary to alter the environment to prevent handicap. Occupational therapists working in social services departments have power to convert front door steps into ramps, install stair lifts, convert baths to showers, and adapt dwellings in whatever way is necessary to suit the particular needs of an inhabitant who has become disabled thus facilitating independence and preventing handicap.

A major problem for people in wheelchairs is mobility within the home. A disabled housewife may be able to work at the sink or transfer from her wheelchair to toilet but these skills are of little use if the kitchen door is too narrow to admit her wheelchair or the hall floor space is too limited to allow her to turn her chair into the bathroom. Good design can anticipate and prevent such handicap.

All local authorities and many housing associations are now building and planning wheelchair bungalows and flats which are specially designed with larger doors, rooms, and circulation space to allow someone who is confined to a wheelchair to move throughout the whole dwelling and use all its facilities. These are specially designed units which are more expensive than conventional dwellings but, as has been emphasized, disabled people are not a separate class in society. Everyone has some functional weakness and bad housing design, for example round, smooth door knobs or modern taps, present difficulties to many people other than those who are severely disabled. Realizing this, architects and designers have shifted their emphasis away from aesthetics and are once more interested in a functional approach, attempting to design an environment that is suitable for people with a very wide range of abilities. The most important example of this trend is the concept of mobility housing which has a number of special features of which the most important is the width of the doors. If housing is built with 900 mm door frames, instead of the 820 mm frames which have been the British standard, those people who use walking aids can move through the doors with ease although the doors look no different and cost is only marginally greater than the conventional door frame. Such housing can accommodate almost all disabled people except those who are permanently in wheelchairs but it looks like ordinary housing and costs little more.

Local authorities and other public bodies now consider disabled people when designing public buildings or considering the plans of private developers. The provision of at least one point of access at ground level, 900 mm wide door frames throughout the building, a toilet suitable for a person in a wheelchair, and lifts, allows disabled people to use colleges, hotels, and council chambers. Even if the problems disabled people face in gaining access to, and moving within, buildings other than their homes are anticipated and precluded, disabled people are often handicapped by their immobility, their inability to move from one building to another.

The mobility problems of disabled people have received widespread publicity in recent years as the Department of Health has shifted its approach from the provision of vehicles to the payment of mobility allowances. These allowances will not completely prevent immobility. They can only mitigate the problem for those who are considered eligible for the weekly payment and they will be of no help to disabled people over pension age because they are not eligible to apply for a mobility allowance. The problem which underlies the handicap of immobility is poverty and for disabled people of working age the main cause of poverty is long-term unemployment. The prevention of unemployment is difficult to achieve by legislation. In spite of the fact that the Employment Medical Advisory Service offers rehabilitation and retraining opportunities, disabled people are frequently unable to find a job even after retraining. It is suggested by the Department of Employment that three per cent of employees should be disabled people, but this has proved impossible to enforce. The employment of disabled people and the primary prevention of poverty probably requires not only a change of employers' attitudes but also a reduction in unemployment rates because the employment prospects of disabled people depend just as much on the state of the whole labour market as on any specific government policy. When unemployment rates are low disabled people stand a chance of employment but in times of recession their chance becomes very slim. Because poverty cannot be prevented by ensuring employment the State has developed a maze of financial benefits for disabled people.

Until recently there were anomalous disparities between the financial benefits given to different groups of disabled people. The amount of money given by the State depended mainly on whether they had become disabled as a result of an injury or disease acquired in the work place or in the armed services, or whether they became disabled as a result of a disease or accident unconnected with work, for example by having been disabled from birth or having developed arthritis while a housewife at home. Those who had become disabled at work or at war received much more generous financial help from the State. However, the introduction of Attendance Allowances for disabled people, Invalid Care Allowances for their supporters, and Non-Contributory Disability Pensions for disabled housewives in the 1970s relieved the poverty which was an all too common consequence of disability. The three allowances introduced in the 1970s were based on a new principle, the need to prevent the handicap of poverty irrespective of the manner in which disability had been acquired. This new approach to the problems of disabled people owed much to the debate aroused by the thalidomide disaster and was discussed in the report of Lord Pearson's *Royal Commission on Civil Liability and Compensation for Personal Injury* which was presented to the Government in 1977. This report endorsed the principle that State compensation for disabled people should judge the person's eligibility for help solely on their disability. The handicap of poverty has been mitigated but not prevented.

In the long run, however, handicaps cannot be prevented by increasing state intervention alone. Only a change in the attitude of members of society towards those who are less able than themselves can bring about the necessary changes.

Mental illness

In 1974, 8 per cent of consultations with general practitioners were recorded as being due to mental disorder. This probably under-estimates the size of the problem, for many people present physical symptoms to their G.P. when the real problem is one of mental upset. The prescription of drugs which affect the mind, psychotropic drugs, has markedly increased over the last decade and one recent study in Oxfordshire found that 9.7 per cent of men and 21.0 per cent of women received at least one prescription for a psychotropic drug each year. This was the average figure; in some age groups the percentage was much higher.

Percentage of people prescribed a psychotropic drug during one year

Age group	Men	Women
15–29	5	16
30–44	12	27
45–59	15	33
60–74	18	32
over 75	27	38

Source: D. C. G. Skegg, R. Doll, and J. Perry, *British Medical Journal* (1977), 1561–1563.

In 1975, more than 175,000 people were admitted to psychiatric hospitals in England—57,000 of them for the first time, the remainder having been admitted in previous years. This means that of every 100,000 men, 314 were admitted to hospital as were 437 of every 100,000 women, the rate of hospital admission in both men and women increasing with age. The cost of mental illness to the N.H.S. is 8 per cent of its total budget, but the total cost to society, in terms of lost productivity, family breakdown, and human misery cannot be calculated.

Before considering the scope for prevention it is necessary to review the prevailing opinions on the nature of mental illness, because it is not unanimously accepted that the conditions called mental illnesses should be dealt with in the same way as are physical illnesses—for example, tonsillitis, cancer, or ischaemic heart disease—that is with doctors as the agents of society who are expected to diagnose, treat, cure, and prevent. There are those who maintain that what is called mental illness is not an illness as such. Some sociologists suggest that many people whom we call mentally ill are merely those who are deviant, who would have been labelled as heretics, criminals, vagrants, or prophets in earlier times. Thomas Szasz, who is himself a professor of psychiatry, is a well-known proponent of this view and the titles of two of his books *The Myth of Mental Illness* and *The Manufacture of Madness* encapsulate his views. R. D. Laing, who is also a psychiatrist, has eloquently claimed, notably in *The Divided Self,* that schizophrenia should not be considered as an illness but as an experience full of meaning and value. Few people accept all the hypotheses of either of these authors, but their views have illuminated the whole field of psychiatry. There is now a consensus that a condition called mental illness exists, but whether it should be regarded as an illness to be treated by doctors, or as a disorder of brain function and behaviour to be managed by psychologists, or as a consequence of difficulties during childhood development to be treated by psychotherapists is not universally agreed. However, the most common type of professional help for people with mental symptoms is a consultation with a doctor and those who consult can be grouped into two categories. There are those whose thought and behaviour is not qualitatively different from the normal range, and those whose mental functioning is abnormal.

The majority of people who attend and are treated by a G.P. have symptoms which everyone experiences—depression, anxiety and tension, sleeplessness—and their symptoms are not qualitatively different from normal. Those who seek medical help are, in general, those who experience more severe symptoms than those who do not consult a doctor, but the severity of symptoms is not the only determining factor. The probability that a person will consult a doctor also depends on his or her alternative means of support. Marriage guidance counsellors, social workers, and Samaritans offer formal alternatives to the G.P. but informal sources of help—

colleagues at work, relatives, and friends — can be equally effective provided an individual has access to them. Men who go out to work or to the pub or who are involved in sporting activities have opportunities to seek informal support no matter where they live but housewives with children may have fewer opportunities. A woman who lives in the same village as her mother and sister, both of whom she loves, and attends the local church will, like anyone else, become depressed and anxious from time to time. She will be less likely to take her problem to her G.P. and be given a prescription for anti-depressant or tranquillizing drugs, however, than if she were a woman living in a new town two hundred miles from her family, neither believing in God nor regularly meeting with any group of people at work or elsewhere.

It can be argued that such alternatives to consultation with the G.P. prevent not mental disturbance but merely the use of health services. However, these informal support systems can also prevent mental problems developing to a level at which they require formal support. For example, a man who can talk over an anxiety with two colleagues at work, who are also friends, and who can then go for a couple of drinks with them to relax and completely dispel his anxiety is continually in receipt of a preventive service, whereas his wife who is at home with their two small children, without a car or friends living nearby, does not have the same opportunities of sharing her problems. The importance of social factors in causing depression in women was clearly demonstrated by G. W. Brown and T. Harris, sociologists working from Bedford College, London, in their study of the *Social Origins of Depression*. Recognition of the fact that depression, anxiety, and other mental symptoms are aggravated by social conditions creates an ethical problem for the medical profession. Is it right to prescribe drugs to damp down such symptoms when the tension which causes them might be able to bring about social changes which would deal with the underlying social problems? Should not doctors strive to change society rather than treating its symptoms? An alternative approach to the prevention of mental symptoms is the development of other means of support, but this is not easy. The secularization of society and its increasing mobility — nearly one household in ten moves every year — diminishes the strength of the social support system and requires people to turn increasingly to professional support.

Changes in society could reduce the number of people who are mentally distressed, for example those depressed by bad housing or poverty, but change itself is a cause of mental disorder which affects people in every class and culture. The plurality of value systems which have replaced the single ethical standard that prevailed in times past makes decision-taking increasingly difficult for individuals who probably experience more episodes of mental disorder in a society which is less supportive.

Some mental disorders are qualitatively different from the normal range of mood and thought. Unlike the previous type of disorder, which was within the normal range although at the extremes of normality, these disorders are abnormal. The commonest type of abnormal mental condition is schizophrenia. Schizophrenia is a complex condition most clearly explained by J. K. Wing in his book *Reasoning about Madness*. The person with schizophrenia is usually affected by delusions, feelings of persecution, irrational thoughts, and absorption in his own thoughts to the exclusion of other people; he is dissociated from family, friends, and society. The search for the cause, or causes, of schizophrenia and other abnormal mental conditions has to focus on both internal factors— the genetic and biochemical constitution of the individual and the way his brain operates—and external factors—his familial, social, and cultural background. Biochemistry, psychology, sociology, psychoanalytic methods, epidemiology, and other approaches have all been used in the study of schizophrenia but the search has been inconclusive and so far the primary prevention of schizophrenia is impossible. However, new treatments have made schizophrenia a less disabling condition, enabling people to live in the community who previously would have been hospitalized for life. Phenothiazine drugs and a therapeutic approach that tries to restore the abilities of the person with schizophrenia to a level which will allow him to return to life in the community can, in combination, prevent the secondary complications of schizophrenia—complete withdrawal from society and dependence on hospital—but the problem of schizophrenia remains unsolved.

Even though schizophrenia is a distinctly abnormal state, easily recognized in its more extreme forms, the boundary between normal and abnormal is often blurred and difficult to define. This is even more difficult when trying to distinguish a normal mood swing from abnormal depression. Everyone experiences periods of depression, some of which can be intense and require treatment by the prescription of anti-depressant drugs if social support is not sufficient. Some people, however, become so severely depressed that they neither eat nor move, and some women cease to menstruate. In some cases no factor can be identified to explain the profound change of mood, and this type of depression is sometimes said to be endogenous in contrast to exogenous depression, which is a normal reaction to a social situation, such as bereavement. In some cases, however, the diagnosis of endogenous depression is made not because there is no cause but because the doctor has been unable to identify it.

Depression is the second commonest reason for admission to psychiatric hospital. Although biochemical disorders have been uncovered in this group of depressed people, no biochemical cause has been identified and prevention is not possible. The secondary effects of depression—suicide, prolonged disability, and hospitalization—can sometimes be prevented by the use of electroconvulsive therapy (E.C.T.) and anti-depressant drugs.

More than half of hospital beds are now occupied by people aged over 65 years. Some of those resident in hospital were admitted as young people with schizophrenia thirty, forty, or more years ago, before phenothiazine drugs were available or an active therapeutic approach employed. However, the major reason why old people are admitted nowadays is dementia, a degeneration of brain tissue which is distinct from the normal process of brain ageing. Some uncommon types of dementia are preventable, for example brain failure due to alcoholism or deficiency of Vitamin B.12, but of the two common types, atherosclerotic dementia and senile dementia, only the former is preventable as the cause of senile dementia is unknown. Only one in six people with dementia live in hospital and they are not necessarily the most severely demented sixth, since admission to hospital is determined not only by the severity of the brain failure but also by social and psychological factors, some of which are preventable. Disturbing behaviour, for example agitation or restlessness, may be difficult to prevent if it is a reflection of the old person's previous personality, but it may be the result of frustration, perhaps caused by unnecessarily locked doors. Thus the behaviour which upsets other people and leads to hospital referral can be prevented by preventing frustration. Isolation from social contacts and deprivation of the sensory stimuli which is received through eyes, ears, and spoken communication can have severe psychological effects such as disorientation in time and space. Someone with dementia is more likely to become isolated and suffer sensory deprivation than an old person whose brain is not failing, and the prevention of isolation and sensory deprivation can prevent further deterioration of mental function. Any type of physical illness can cause mental disorder in old age, but an old person with dementia who develops a physical illness may not be able to explain her symptoms to other people who may ascribe them as being due to her dementia. Careful medical supervision can prevent unnecessary mental deterioration, but treatment must be cautious because people with dementia are very sensitive to drugs and problems often arise from drug side-effects which could have been prevented by more careful prescribing and supervision. The members of a family looking after a disabled old person also need support whether they are married children, single sons or daughters—more than 300,000 single children care for elderly parents— or other relatives. This applies as much to families caring for people disabled by dementia as it does to those caring for people with schizophrenia. Family breakdown often leads to hospital admission which may be preventable by the early and sympathetic use of support services, such as the incontinent laundry service, or hospital admission to allow the supporters to go on holiday.

Mental illness presents preventive medicine with its most subtle and difficult challenge.

Prevention of absence from work through sickness

The loss of working days due to sickness absence is always much greater than those lost as a result of strikes, yet sickness absence rarely hits the headlines. It was calculated in 1971 that the total cost of sickness—national insurance payments, lost earnings, and lost productivity—was equal to the cost of running the National Health Service. Sickness absence is a major economic issue as well as being a challenge to preventive medicine.

The sickness absence figures collected by the Department of

Health and Social Security have to be interpreted with caution because there are some minor inaccuracies, for example spells of absence of less than three days duration are not notified, and the sickness rates in the armed forces are not included. The categories of disease responsible for sickness absence reflect the pattern of disease seen by the G.P. in his consulting room. These figures, however, include both short-term and long-term absences which should be considered separately.

Percentage of total work days lost in England and Wales

19 ••••••••••••••••••	Respiratory infections, bronchitis and asthma
10•••••••••••	Mental illness
9 •••••••••	Accidents
7 ••••••••	Arthritis and rheumatism
6 ••••••	Ischaemic heart disease
6 ••••••	Digestive disorders

Source: D. F. K. Black and J. D. Pole, *British Journal of Social and Preventive Medicine* (1975), 29:222–227.

Prevention of short-term absence

The General Household Survey found that people who were satisfied with their work were less frequently off sick than those who were dissatisfied. This finding is not surprising. The decision on whether or not to take a symptom to a doctor is influenced by many factors. The severity of the symptom, the results of self-treatment, and the advice of others, are all important but so are the rewards which may follow as a result of becoming ill. To become ill is not only a change in a person's physical condition, it is a change in his social condition. Being ill has certain rewards—the right to be excused normal obligations such as work and the right to receive sympathy— but they are given only to those whose illness is accepted by society and to be excused work usually requires a doctor's statement that the illness is genuine. Someone who is a self-employed craftsman doing a job he loves will probably continue to work even though he develops the symptoms of a cold. If, however, the same man were working on a noisy production line doing a tiring and boring job in uncongenial surroundings he might well consult his doctor with the same degree of symptoms, not so much for a diagnosis or treatment, but to be validated as being sick and thus obtain relief from his job in a manner acceptable to his employers and work-mates. The prevention of sickness absence, is therefore more a matter for management and unions than one for the medical profession.

In a firm in which job satisfaction is low, sickness absence is more common than in a similar firm in which job satisfaction is higher. Short-term absence is not only the end result of the physical and mental symptoms experienced by employees, it is itself a symptom of the employee's social well-being, his feeling of satis-faction. Firms in which short-term sickness is high also often have production problems—both with respect to the quantity and to the quality of work done—and a high rate of staff turnover. Job satisfaction is obviously impaired if workers are paid less than the rate they regard as fair for the type of work done, and if the physical conditions in which they work are unpleasant. However, high wages and good working conditions alone do not ensure job satis-faction, although it is difficult to achieve if they are not present. The more important influences are social and psychological. The intrinsic nature of the job itself obviously affects the attitudes of employees but, irrespective of this, satisfaction with any type of work can be enhanced if the individual is given freedom in the organization of his work, opportunity to experiment and use skill, the ability to identify with the end product, recognition and reward for achievement, the chance of promotion, and other opportunities to express his individuality through work. All these are easier to offer in a small organization but even a larger concern can scale down its operations into small semi-autonomous units, groups with which an individual can identify and in which the motivating factors can be developed. Technology sometimes necessitates large-scale production lines, for example to make low-cost motor cars. The social problems in car factories are well-known. Volvo have moved away from the production line to allow teams to build complete cars but this technique is inapplicable to the construction of low-cost cars. Another approach has been to instal complete automation of the line, as has been attempted in Japan and America, but this may merely replace one form of industrial disease with another—unemployment.

For many years employers complained that general practitioners wrote sickness certificates too readily, little realizing that G.P.s were themselves dissatisfied on a number of grounds. Doctors appreciated that they were frequently unaware of a man's working conditions and the nature of his job; they were aware of the fact that social conditions at work could influence an individual's behaviour and were sometimes in sympathy with someone's unconscious desire to have a few day's respite; and they did not believe that they had studied medicine to act as unpaid controllers of those people who sought relief from uncongenial work. There were frequent calls for the complete abolition of the system of certification. These have been resisted but, as a concession, the Department of Health and Social Security changed the term 'Doctor's Certificate' to 'Doctor's Statement' in 1976. The G.P. is no longer expected to certify someone as being just unfit, he issues a statement recording his advice about refraining from work. This is a subtle but important change but many G.P.s are still unhappy about the effect on the doctor-patient relationship which would result if they were to investigate every request for a sickness certificate with rigour and thoroughness. Short-term sickness absence can only be prevented if both medical and social causes are tackled. Some employers immunize their employees against influenza, although the benefits of this policy are not agreed by everyone, but increasingly employers and personnel officers recognize that the social factors are the most important.

Prevention of long-term sickness absence

Social factors also influence long-term sickness absence. In a survey of people off sick for six months, the diseases responsible were similar to those responsible for disability in the Amelia Harris survey (see page 86).

The length of time a person stays off work is affected by the nature of his occupation in long-term sickness absences as in short-term absence. In the survey cited it was found, not surprisingly, that those who were in physically demanding jobs had to stay off longer than those who were in light office jobs. It was also those who were off sick from less-skilled jobs who were less frequently covered by sick pay and more frequently lost their jobs as a result of

Principal causes of long-term sickness absence 1972/73

Percentage of people off work for six months	Type of disease
31 ••••••••••••••••••••••••••••••••	Heart and circulatory
18 ••••••••••••••••••	Bone and joint
17 •••••••••••••••••	Respiratory
16 ••••••••••••••••	Results of accidents
12 ••••••••••••	Mental
10 ••••••••••	Digestive

Source: J. Martin and M. Morgan. *Prolonged sickness absence and the return to work.* Office of Population Censuses and Survey, Social Surveys division (H.M.S.O., 1975).

their sickness absence. The consequence of this was that they sometimes not only became unemployed but also, because the causes of long-term sickness absence occur in middle age and often have permanent effects, virtually unemployable. The research workers were emphatic in their conclusion that 'it does not seem from our results that lack of motivation to return to work in itself causes sickness to be prolonged. The long-term sick seemed to want to return to work but the practical problems many faced frequently made their return extremely difficult.'

Prevention of industrial disease

Working conditions can also cause illness directly. Very unsatisfactory conditions can cause mental disorder which becomes manifest either as mental symptoms or as physical symptoms of psychosomatic type, such as headaches. Working conditions can also cause physical disorders by the exposure of a worker to noxious materials or to the risk of accident. Under the National Insurance (Industrial Injuries) Act of 1946 a number of diseases were prescribed which could be caused as a result of working conditions. The purpose of this list and the conditions specified for each disease was to clarify eligibility for injury and disablement benefits. Tuberculosis, for instance, is a prescribed disease, but industrial injury benefit is payable only if the disease has been acquired in the professional care of an affected person, or in the course of laboratory investigation of tuberculosis, or if the infection occurred as a result of research work using material which carries the infection. Other examples of disease prescribed under the industrial injuries scheme are poisoning by lead, mercury, or arsenic; anthrax, from the handling of wool, hair, bristles, hides, and skins; mesothelioma from asbestos; Farmer's Lung (see page 105); and bladder cancer caused by naphthylamine (see page 69). A full list of prescribed industrial diseases is included in Department of Health leaflet NI 2. There are separate leaflets for pneumoconiosis (see page 105) and occupational deafness, leaflets NI 3 and NI 201 respectively.

Sickness absence resulting from the prescribed diseases is very much less than sickness absence caused by diseases which have no causal connection with working conditions. In the years from 1968 to 1972 the average number of days lost each year from certified sickness was 17,160 for every 1,000 members of the working population. By comparison, over the same period only 47 days were lost annually because of prescribed diseases per 1,000 workers. Insignificant though this appears to be, these prescribed diseases are extremely important not only because they are preventable but because of their symbolic significance. The principles which underlie the contract between employer and employee have been codified in the last one hundred-and-fifty years by a succession of Parliamentary Acts. A framework of legislation has been built to protect the employee from danger at work, to treat him if he fell ill, and to compensate him if he sustained injury, illness, or permanent disability in the course of his employment. As the trade union movement grew in power and authority it emphasized that illness was frequently contracted in the financial interest of others whose attempts to minimize production costs, in order to increase their return on capital, often increased the risk to which their employees were exposed. The Factory Act of 1844 included clauses on safety for the first time and it provided two schemes for workers' compensation in both of which the state had a role to play. The principle of liability without fault, that is that it was unnecessary to prove the employers' negligence to obtain compensation was not established until the Workmen's Compensation Act of 1897 which remained in force until the Industrial Injuries Act of 1946.

The range of diseases acquired through work are as varied as the nature of work itself. Chemical substances can cause disease, both inorganic chemicals such as arsenic, lead, chromium, and cadmium, and organic compounds. If the chemical is in the form of the gas it can readily cause disease as the inhalation of gas exposes the lungs directly to chemical damage. The noxious factor may be physical, for example radioactive material or noise. The effect produced depends not only on the particular noxious qualities of the agent concerned but also on the duration and intensity of exposure, the manner of contact, whether the substance is inhaled, swallowed, or absorbed through the skin, and the response of the individual, for not all people respond identically to the same stimulus. People may also acquire infections at work, not only from their colleagues who may transmit influenza or other illnesses which could be caught away from work, but from some jobs which carry their own peculiar risks of infection. Veterinary surgeons not infrequently acquire brucellosis, and staff working in renal dialysis units may acquire hepatitis.

Three main types of industrial disease dominate the picture: skin disease, lung disease, and cancer. Occupational dermatitis is responsible for the loss of over 850,000 working days every year— more days than are lost from all the other prescribed industrial diseases added together. Dermatitis can be caused by mechanical trauma, such as friction; physical factors such as heat, cold, or radiation, inorganic and organic chemical agents; and plant or other biological material such as insects. Often these factors act in concert, but chemical dermatitis is the most common. Much of the economic and social cost of occupational skin disease is preventable.

There are two main types of lung disease. Allergic lung disease is caused by the inhalation of biological protein which can result in asthma (see page 76) or a diffuse type of inflammation, and a large number of such inflammatory diseases have been described, for example Farmer's Lung which is caused by the inhalation of the spores of *Thermoactinomyces vulgaris* which multiply in mouldy hay. Pneumoconiosis is the other more important type of lung disease. It is caused by the deposition of dust in the lung tissue, the most common dusts being carbon and silicon. Although dust is now much better controlled in coal mines, quarries, and iron foundries about 1,000 new cases are still notified every year and more than 40,000 people continue to receive benefit because they are disabled by pneumoconiosis. In mining areas it is a major cause of long-term sickness absence and unemployment.

Cancer can be caused by the work environment. Skin cancer can be caused by pitch and tar; bladder cancer by certain chemicals (see page 69); lung cancer by nickel, chromates, and asbestos; and leukaemia by radiation. Industrial cancers are uncommon but they are a grim and constant reminder that any new chemical compound has to be regarded with the suspicion that it could be a carcinogen and treated with caution because its effects, if it has any, may not become evident until it has been in use for years (see page 173).

A number of options are open to the employer whose employees are exposed to risk. He can substitute a substance which is not toxic for the one which is, for example other fire-resistant material is now used in place of asbestos. Alternatively, he can completely enclose the material and its processing, as radioactive material is handled remotely, or he can try to minimize the exposure of the individual to the toxic phase of the process by extracting fumes or dust at the site of production. The principle underlying these approaches is that they do not rely on the employee's co-operation. Even though protective masks, gloves, clothes, and hats are given to a worker for his own protection, he may not wear them if they are uncomfortable, or slow his work rate and reduce his pay. The prevention of industrial disease depends on the actions of employer and employee, and the way in which they act is determined by their attitudes. Those of the individual employee are influenced by the attitudes of other workers and of the management staff. If the union or employee's organization demands in-service training and the provision of protective clothing, and if management not only responds but initiates other preventive measures, the individual will be more likely to be safety conscious than if both are indifferent.

The social environment is of even greater importance in the prevention of accidents. There are nearly half-a-million accidents at work every year, of which about 1,000 are fatal. The term 'accident' is misleading in its implication that chance or fortune are important factors. In fact cause and effect can often be clearly identified and many accidents are preventable. The Factory Inspectorate undertook a study of a number of accidents in a sample of 46 factories of different types. Their conclusion was that the most important preventive influence was the attitude of management. Some occupations are obviously more hazardous than others, but firms doing the same type of work were compared and it was discovered that those in which there is only token consultation between management and staff, in which too much emphasis is placed on the collection of statistics in lieu of action, and in which top management is uninterested in accident prevention, had a higher rate of accidents, both fatal and non-fatal. In those factories in which top management committed themselves to accident prevention in word and action there was not only a lower rate of accidents but higher productivity, lower sickness absence, and lower labour turnover. Prominence is given to the dangers of mining, but miners and mine managers are very safety conscious. Much of the credit must go to the actions of the National Union of Mine Workers which is in turn based on the tightly knit social cohesion of mining communities. By comparison the record of the construction industry is very much worse, reflecting the less well organized, more mobile, unstable nature of the industry and its work-force.

Although the present level of sickness absence and industrial disease leaves much to be desired, a great deal of sound preventive medicine has been practised at work. The level of illness would be very much higher if it were not for the network of monitoring and inspecting activities which have been developed in the last century-and-a-half through legislation. The prevention of illness related to work will be extremely difficult. Each year sees the production of an ever-increasing number of new compounds and each of these compounds has a number of residues, the possible harmful effects of which may not become evident until years after workers were first exposed to them. The prevention of industrial disease requires the closest inspection of every new process, the awareness of the social factors which influence the way workers react to the protective measures provided for them, and a balanced programme of education and legislation (see page 167).

Hidden challenges

There are certain common, and serious, problems which are not revealed by the statistics of mortality and morbidity discussed so far. Obesity, dental decay, problems caused by alcohol, and the ageing of the population do not appear among the common causes of death, disability, G.P. consultations, sickness absence from

work, or any other of the commonly used measures of the state of
the public health but they present major challenges to prevention.

Obesity

Obese people have higher mortality rates than those who are not
obese, but just how great the risk of obesity may be is difficult to
determine because other risk factors, such as cigarette smoking,
complicate the calculations. There is enough evidence to convince
actuaries, however, and insurance premiums are increased for
obese people. The greater the weight of the person who wishes to
be insured when compared with the average for people of the same
sex, age, and height as himself, the higher the premium. For
example, the Mercantile and General underwriting manual which
is a standard work in the insurance world, suggests a 10 per cent
loading on men 1.83m (6 feet) tall who are 5 per cent above the
average weight, a 30 per cent increase for those 30 per cent over
weight, and a 50 per cent increase for those 40 per cent over the
average.

Obesity predisposes to and complicates many illnesses. Although
the relationship of obesity to heart disease is uncertain (see page 64)
there is no doubt that it predisposes to osteoarthritis, herniae,
varicose veins, gallstones, certain types of diabetes, gout, high
blood pressure and other diseases. Obesity makes surgery more
difficult and operative and post-operative complications are more
probable in obese people.

Obesity is apparently simple to cure, requiring only a reduced
intake of energy, but many people find this difficult to achieve and
therefore demand appetite suppressant drugs. In 1975, £3.5 million
worth of appetite suppressant drugs were prescribed, although the
British National Formulary, one of the medical profession's official
drug guides, pronounced that 'there is no substitute for will-power'.
G.P.s and health visitors attempt to help those who do not have
sufficient will-power to lose weight on their own by means other
than the prescription of drugs, by organizing slimming clubs or
seeing and encouraging the individual at regular intervals. School
doctors and nurses employ the same methods in schools but failure
is common. Weight Watchers and other self-help groups manage
to support some people whom the professionals cannot help.

Although the motives of those who attend such groups are as frequently aesthetic as they are salutory, the loss in weight which many members achieve is beneficial to their health. Exercise, an increase in the energy expenditure, is much less effective than decreased energy intake over a short period of time as a means of losing weight, but it can contribute to the long term control of body weight if it is taken regularly, in addition to its other benefits (see page 64). To encourage this approach to obesity the 'Look After Yourself' campaign, launched by the Health Education Council and Scottish Health Education Unit in 1978, emphasized the need to combine regular exercise with a prudent diet, one which is low in fat and sugar and high in fibre.

Although obesity has its dangers, dieting is not without risk. Just how common anorexia nervosa is, and whether it has increased in recent years, is uncertain but it is more frequently reported by many people working with adolescents. Anorexia nervosa is, of course, not just an exaggeration of normal dieting, being a manifestation of a profound psychological disturbance, but it is possible that disturbed adolescents girls develop anorexia rather than some other disorder because of the associated images of slimness and attractiveness which prevail in modern society.

Dental decay

Recent evidence shows that dental decay is now the most common chronic disease in Europe. By the age of 15 the average child has 17 of his 28 permanent teeth decayed, filled, or missing, and more than 7,000 dentures are supplied to school children every year. In 1968 a survey in England and Wales found that 38 per cent of people over the age of 16 had had all their teeth extracted and the proportion was 44 per cent in Scotland. Dental disease costs the N.H.S. £200 million annually and is responsible for the loss of 4 million working days. It is a huge problem. Dental decay and periodontal (gum) disease, which is a common reason for extraction in older people, has become more common because of a change in dietary habits, principally the increase in the intake of purified carbohydrate, sugar, which has taken place during the last century.

The mainstay of prevention is the education of children and their parents. Each area health authority has a dental health education service which co-operates with the education authority to provide education in schools. In 1975, 23,000 dental health education sessions were held throughout Britain, most of them in schools but a proportion for the mothers of children under school age. The General Dental Council and the British Dental Association have produced health education material in co-operation with the Health Education Council and Scottish Health Education Unit, both of which have dental health education advisory groups. The emphasis of education is to warn parents and children of the dangers of sugar, and to help people keep their teeth clean to prevent the formation of bacterial plaque, the cause of dental decay. Dental hygienists and dental auxiliaries, who receive less training than dentists and are therefore less expensive, help in prevention by reinforcing dental health education. They also remove the more resistant plaque periodically in treatment sessions which are primarily preventive.

The House of Commons Expenditure Sub-Committee (see page 115) recommended that more dental hygienists be trained and employed, but the government in the White Paper, *Prevention and Health,* only accepted this 'with reservations'. Reservations were also expressed on the recommendations that fissure sealants, a plastic coating applied to the teeth then hardened by ultraviolet light, and direct fluoride applications be made available on the N.H.S. because the benefits of these techniques are thought to be little more effective than the regular brushing of teeth in the correct manner with fluoride toothpaste, while their cost is very much greater than self-help. The White Paper stated that the department of health 'did not feel justified at present, however, in advising more extended use (of fissure sealing and fluoride applications) but prefer to encourage authorities to introduce the fluoridation of water supplies'. Fluoridation is indubitably the cheapest and most effective method of preventing dental decay. It is safe and comparatively simple to add to drinking water at the waterworks yet, by the end of 1975, no more than 9 per cent of the population of the United Kingdom received water containing one part per million of fluoride, the necessary level to prevent caries. The resistance to fluoridation on both ethical and factual grounds having been entrenched for many years, the dental profession asked the Royal College of Physicians to review the evidence on the beneficial and harmful effects of fluoride in 1973. The report *Fluoride Teeth and Health*, published in 1976, stated categorically that 'there is no evidence that fluoridation has any harmful effect' but even this unequivocal endorsement for the safety of fluoride did little or nothing to influence the opponents of fluoridation. Aware of the groundswell of suspicion and opposition, the government in its White Paper *Prevention and Health* merely stated that 'it would continue to promote the general introduction of fluoridation of water supplies', but even so gave no indication of whether it was prepared to take any more effective action. It seems unlikely that a government would take legislative action on this issue unless it had a large majority, and the main emphasis of preventive dentistry in future, as at present, will be educative.

Alcohol abuse

In the year 81 A.D. the Emperor Dominian decreed that half the vineyards in Britain be laid waste to prevent the problems caused by the excessive consumption of wine. Since then the problems caused by alcohol have been a permanent feature in Britain and all European countries. In the last twenty years the problems have increased at an alarming rate. There has been an increase in drunken driving (see page 80); drunkenness convictions have doubled since 1955; short-term absence from work due to hangovers and drunkenness has increased; and crimes precipitated by alcohol, such as wife and child battering, have also increased. These acute problems are the results of heavy drinking sessions, but there is evidence of a similar rate of increase in the problems caused by the chronic consumption of excessive amounts of alcohol, for example the death rate from liver cirrhosis increased by 50 per cent between 1955 and 1975, and other physical illnesses caused by alcohol have also increased. In addition to its damaging physical effects alcohol causes physical dependence, with the result that an individual suffers physical symptoms such as 'the shakes' when he stops drinking, and psychological dependence, with the result that he cannot stop drinking, a combination usually called alcoholism. Alcohol taken over long periods can cause mental illness, called alcoholic psychosis, but the distinction between this and alcoholism is not clear-cut and they are usually considered together. The rate of admission to psychiatric hospitals for these two conditions increased by about 50 per cent between 1970 and 1975. The physical, mental, and social consequences of chronic alcohol abuse can occur in any combination and appear in any guise, from an individual whose only problem is cirrhosis to someone who has a whole range of physical illnesses, who is psychotic, and who sleeps rough or in a Cyrenians hostel having dropped out from his family and culture. The acute and chronic problems are interrelated. Those people who are serious drinking and driving offenders, and those who batter their wives and children are frequently people with a chronic serious drink problem, not just individuals who have indulged on one occasion.

Particularly worrying is the rate of increase of both acute and chronic problems among women and young people between 1965 and 1975. Offences of drunkenness in the age group 18–21 increased by 90 per cent in males, and 400 per cent in females. The effects of alcohol often precipitate otherwise well-balanced young people into crime—stealing cars, breaking and entering, and crimes of violence—and alcohol, by anaesthetising the inhibitions of young girls, can lead to unwanted pregnancies and venereal disease.

It may be that the rate of increase is slowing. The total number of proved offences of drunkenness and the number of proceedings against motorists in England and Wales in 1977 were fewer than in 1976, and the same trend was revealed in Scotland. Whether this represents a real decrease in the number of such problems caused by alcohol or whether it is rather caused by changing patterns of police work or of consumer expenditure, due to a decrease in the real value of incomes, or by some other social trend, requires further data to determine. However, such changes, if they are real, will have little effect on the official estimate that there are currently about 500,000 people with a serious drink problem, and this presents a major problem for prevention (see page 165).

Problems of old age

Although many elderly people are active and independent until the end of their lives, some are disabled by disease and become dependent. Disability occurs with increasing frequency as age advances, and people aged over 75 make heavy demands on the health and social services, although it must be emphasized that the majority in this age group are independent. The number of people aged over 75 will increase by more than 500,000 by 1995, which will pose considerable problems to health and social services; but some of their difficulties can be prevented.

It is important to distinguish between the effects of ageing, which is a normal biological process, and the effects of having lived in a certain environment with a certain life style for a long period of time. The ageing process is not preventable but many of the diseases of old age are caused by the previous habits and environment of elderly people. For example, bronchitis is common in old age but this is caused not by lung or bronchial ageing but by the effects of six decades of life in polluted air. Heart disease is common in old age and may be due to ageing of heart tissue, but it may also be the result of the individual's cigarette smoking or dietary intake of fat during the previous fifty years. The prevention of all the other disorders discussed so far can therefore prevent some of the disease and disability in old age. Even when disease occurs as a part of the ageing process its consequences can sometimes be prevented. For example, osteoporosis, the thinning of bones which makes them more fragile, appears to be a consequence of normal ageing. Osteoporosis cannot be prevented but some falls and fractures may be preventable if the home environment of old people is made safer (see page 83).

Sometimes ageing and life-style interact. For example, osteo-arthritis, which is apparently a result of ageing (see page 89), is aggravated by obesity which is a consequence of a certain life-style.

The social problems which so frequently follow medical problems in old age are equally important. Bad housing, heating problems (which may lead to hypothermia), poverty, and isolation are serious but soluble problems, if society wishes to solve them. Prevention of the problems which may occur in old age should start in youth but many people do not consider old age until they retire. Pre-retirement education, which is still in its infancy, is the first line of prevention but it is now reinforced by other educational opportunities for retired people and, increasingly, by the activities of elderly people themselves.

When disability occurs G.P.s, health visitors, home help organizers, district nurses, social and voluntary workers can prevent serious problems, but it has been clearly demonstrated by Sir Ferguson Anderson and James Williamson, professors of geriatric medicine in Glasgow and Edinburgh, that the prevention of problems in old age requires professional and voluntary services to seek out problems at an early stage. Waiting for disabled elderly people to ask for help may mean that the problem, or problems, are insoluble and very difficult to alleviate by the time the professional is asked for help. An old person, her family, and even her professional advisers may accept failing vision as being 'due to old age' and not seek help until glaucoma, a treatable eye disease, has reached a stage at which the damage is irreversible. Similarly, an elder may assume that loss of hearing is due to the normal process of ageing and postpone seeking help until she has become deaf, isolated, withdrawn, and unable to learn how to lip read or use a hearing aid.

In 1978 The Department of Health and Social Security and the Welsh Office issued *A Discussion Document on Elderly People in Our Society—A Happier Old Age* stimulating comment for a White Paper in 1979. The theme of this paper was hopeful, emphasizing that although some of the problems which can occur in old age were inevitable and required good health and social services, many were preventable. To prevent poverty would require a massive investment, but some problems could be prevented by lesser investment in such services as those providing artificial pacemakers or artificial hips (see page 89). To prevent some common problems many people could be helped by comparatively small increases in health and social services. The expansion of the chiropody services could prevent not only disorders of the feet but isolation, and those problems which are consequences of isolation, such as failure to eat an adequate diet, and mental disorder.

6 Ways and means

Legislation

The scope of legislation

Because the public's health is influenced by such fundamental
factors as a nation's wealth, its style of distributive justice, and the
priority it accords to basic services such as the provision of water
and sanitation, there is no branch of government which is not
involved in the prevention of disease (see page 19). Even the
Ministry of Defence influences the public health; positively by
giving employment, negatively by consuming resources which
could be spent directly on prevention and treatment. Even if the
term preventive medicine is narrowed to embrace only those policies
which are primarily designed to prevent premature death and
disease many central government departments are involved. The
Departments of Education and Science, Prices and Consumer
Protection, Employment, and the Environment, the Ministry of
Agriculture, Fisheries and Food, and the Home Office are all
involved, as well as the Department of Health and the ubiquitous,
inscrutable Treasury. Recognizing the complexity of the administrative framework and the importance of prevention, back-bench
M.P.s, members of the all-party Social Services and Employment
Sub-Committee of the House of Commons Expenditure Committee,
began an inquiry into preventive medicine in 1975. They considered
evidence from many sources and published a report in 1977
stimulating a quick, but thorough, response from the Departments
of Health and Education which, together with the Welsh and
Scottish Offices, presented the White Paper 'Prevention and Health'
to the House of Commons in December of the same year. The
responsible Departments were more cautious than the back-
benchers but they accepted 25 of the 66 recommendations made by

the Employment and Social Services Sub-Committee without qualification, and they accepted 17 of them with reservations. Only 8 were rejected outright, the remaining 16 being said to have been 'under consideration' when the White Paper was presented.

Laws can be used to control individuals, to prevent them behaving in ways which are known to increase the probability of illness. Legislation may be directly prohibitory, for example by prohibiting motor cycle riding unless the rider wears a crash helmet. There is strong ethical opposition to this type of legislation (see page 156). Except in these cases in which the intention is to protect children from the consequences of their actions, such as the legal prohibition on the sale of alcohol to young people under 18 years of age and the sale of tobacco to those under 16 years, it can be criticized as being too paternalistic. Although there is ethical opposition to direct legal control of behaviour, the law exerts many indirect controls on behaviour for the benefit of the individual who is controlled.

Prevention through taxation

Taxes have been levied on goods for centuries but the role of taxation has until recently been fiscal, to raise revenue for the Exchequer, and protective, to safeguard native agriculture, trade, and industry—it has not been concerned with the prevention of disease. Her Majesty's Commissioners of Customs and Excise have played a central part in such taxation for more than 600 years, Geoffrey Chaucer was a Controller of Customs in 1374, and as free trade has increased over the last hundred years, the function of the Commissioners has become increasingly orientated towards fiscal objectives, helping to raise the increasing amounts of wealth required by the state to pay for the steadily growing range of activities funded by public expenditure (see page 21). This is a more difficult process than it appears at first sight. An increase in taxation on alcohol and tobacco will certainly increase the amount of revenue obtained from each item sold, but the rise in price will also inhibit demand and may reduce the total amount sold. The amount by which the tax is increased must be carefully calculated to ensure that the decrease in demand and sales will not be so great as to reduce the total amount of revenue collected. The technique used to calculate the appropriate tax increase to supply the necessary revenue is known as demand analysis. Consumers have learned to anticipate the Chancellor's actions and recent years have seen a boom in pre-Budget purchasing of alcohol and tobacco followed by a temporary post-Budget slump before the demand picks up once more, as people become accustomed to the higher price. The demand for alcohol and tobacco is affected not only by the price of these commodities in money terms but by their price in relative terms, that is in comparison to the price of other goods, and by their price in real terms, that is in comparison to the amount of work which has to be done to earn enough money to buy, for example, a bottle of whisky or twenty cigarettes (see page 166). This is well-illustrated by the levels of consumption of alcohol and tobacco in Britain which rose steadily after the Second World War in spite of successive increases in taxation and what appeared to be a tremendous increase in the price of both commodities. This increase was, however, only an increase in money terms; in both relative and real terms the price of these goods did not increase so dramatically, in fact the real price of cigarettes fell in the years of apparent prosperity between 1968 and 1974. Realizing this the Cabinet decided in 1974 to increase the price of cigarettes in real terms and to ensure that the increase in tax was sufficient in magnitude to depress demand. Between March 1974 and April 1977 taxation more than doubled in money terms, and, although the increase in real terms was substantially less, this seems to have been a crucial factor in the reduction of the demand for cigarette tobacco. The Chancellor of the Exchequer became a health minister and the indirect taxation of Customs and Excise duty developed a preventive role.

Having accepted the principle that taxation should be used as a form of preventive medicine it was possible to take discriminatory action against certain types of tobacco. In the Budget in March 1977 the Chancellor increased the tax on cigarettes and hand-rolling tobacco for the fifth successive Budget, telling the Commons that there were 'compelling health reasons' for his move. However, he spared other tobacco products such as pipe tobacco which is much less noxious and, he said, 'plays an important part in the life of many retired people'. One year later the same Chancellor, Mr. Healey, imposed a supplementary tax on high tar cigarettes, again making his intention quite plain:

The House will recognize that this supplementary duty is not designed primarily to raise revenue—it could bring in only £25m. in a full year at most—and if it results in leading smokers to abandon these high tar cigaretes, no one will be more pleased than I.

The Employment and Social Services Sub-Committee's report recommended that 'an increase in duty to achieve a price increase sufficient to reduce cigarette consumption should be imposed annually', but the White Paper was more cautious because it maintained that some smokers least able to afford tobacco 'may forego necessities' if the price was increased considerably and that the effect of such taxes on the retail price index might affect 'wage negotiations and hence the general management of the economy'. The only promise made in the White Paper was that the 'Government will continue to consider this recommendation'. Whatever happens, it is unlikely that the price of cigarettes will ever again be allowed to fall in real terms as it did between 1968 and 1974. Taxation is now an integral part of the campaign against cigarette smoking.

The demand for alcohol is also influenced by its price, relative to the price of other goods and to its real value, in terms of the labour required to purchase it. Between 1970 and 1976 the price of beer fell by 4 per cent, that of wine by 14 per cent, and that of spirits by 21 per cent compared with the retail price index, that is the relative price decreased, and the average disposable income increased by 17 per cent in real terms over the same period thus decreasing the real price of alcohol. The Employment and Social Services Sub-Committee recommended that the price of alcohol be maintained at the same level relative to both prices and income, but the Government, in its White Paper, did not accept this recommendation. It was rejected for the same reasons that the Government gave for their caution over cigarette taxation, principally its fear of the general economic implications of price increases. It did not reject the suggestion out of hand, however. The proposal is under consideration and the White Paper stated that 'Health Ministers wish to encourage public debate' on this issue (see page 166).

Legal limits to availability

Another indirect control is that imposed by the limited availability of tobacco, alcohol, and other drugs. Tobacco is widely available to adults but it is an offence for a retailer to sell cigarettes to persons under the age of 16. However, this presents little obstacle to a young person who can purchase cigarettes from a vending machine. The Employment and Social Services Sub-Committee recommended that vending machines should be restricted to premises to which young people under the age of 16 were not admitted. The Government rejected this proposal because it required new legislation, preferring to urge the owners of machines that they be supervised effectively. The availability of alcohol is controlled by licensing laws which are the responsibility of magistrates and the Home Office. The number of licensed premises has increased over the last fifty years, the most significant figures being the increases in the number of clubs and off-licences. The proliferation of off-licences causes most anxiety to those concerned by the increase in alcohol-related problems. The increase is particularly marked among women and young people (see page 111), and it is possible that self-service and supermarket off-licences have increased the availability of alcohol to these groups. The number of hours which each licensed premises is open is also determined by the licensing courts but the influence on drinking habits of different patterns of opening times is uncertain. If licensed premises were opened for longer periods people would probably consume more alcohol, but they might also drink in a more controlled and moderate fashion, so the overall effect of increasing licensing hours is unpredictable. There is, however, unanimous agreement that the minimum legal age for the purchase and consumption of alcohol should not be reduced below 18 years of age. These matters have received considerable consideration at national level, but at magistrates licensing courts the decision on whether or not to grant another off-licence or to extend opening hours is usually considered not in terms of prevention but in terms of trade, and the opposition to proposals for new licences is usually made by those who fear their trade will be affected rather than by those who wish to prevent alcohol abuse.

The availability of other drugs is limited by the Misuse of Drugs Act 1971. Some drugs, for example amphetamines and barbiturates, can be legally possessed by members of the public if they have been prescribed by a doctor but others, for example pethidine and morphine, are almost always administered by nurses or doctors so that the drug is available only when it is medically indicated and administered, although the Act allows specially licensed medical practitioners to prescribe these drugs for addicts, provided that the addicted persons have been notified to the Home Office. Further control is applied by the Customs and Excise Act 1952 which regulates the import and export of such drugs. Tight legal controls prevent some problems but they also create others: the right conditions for a black market for anyone willing to run the risk, and the crimes which inevitably follow black markets. Such controls also alienate any section of the community which does not agree with the state's definition that a drug is dangerous and a number of young people have lost respect for the law as a result of their treatment by police and courts after they have been arrested for the possession of cannabis (see page 158).

Prevention through the traditional role of law

The use of the law to protect people from the harmful consequences of their own actions is controversial on ethical grounds (see page 156); the law is on a much firmer and more traditional footing when it is used to protect individuals from harm resulting from the activities of other people. Most of the legislation which was drafted and enacted to prevent disease is based on this principle. It can be considered in five main classes; the laws relating to road safety (see page 77); those covering health and safety at work (see page 168); those which are concerned with environmental health and the prevention of infectious disease; those intended to prevent death from fire; and those laws which set standards for food, drugs, and other consumer goods.

The keystone of environmental health legislation is the Public Health Act of 1936. There are 347 sections in this amending and consolidating Act which repealed Acts as diverse as the Baths and Wash-houses Act of 1846 and the Public Health (Prevention and Treatment of Disease) Act 1913 and embraced Acts as varied as the Rivers Pollution Prevention Act 1876 and the Infectious Disease (Prevention) Act of 1890. The Act was drafted as a public health charter covering drains and sewers; water supply; nuisances, for example smoke and offensive trades, such as fat extraction or glue making; the prevention, identification, and treatment of disease; the provision of hospitals; and maternal and child welfare. Some of these sections were repealed by subsequent legislation, but those which covered environmental health still provide the basis on which laws covering modern environmental hazards are drafted, although the framework is being increasingly altered by the incorporation of E.E.C. regulations (see page 172).

Death from fire evokes a strong emotional response, especially when a number of people die simultaneously, but deaths can be precluded by preventing fire from starting, slowing the spread of fires throughout buildings and ensuring the detection of a fire at an early stage thus allowing people more time to escape. The Department of the Environment and local housing authorities are responsible for enforcing the regulations which cover multi-occupied dwellings, but all other premises are controlled by Acts emanating from the Home Office and implemented by local fire authorities. Certain Acts cover licensing and gaming premises, others cover places of entertainment, with the Fire Precautions Act 1971 as the mainstay of legislation.

In the control of food and drug standards the Food and Drugs Act of 1955 stands in an analogous position to the Public Health Act 1936. It is of central importance, consolidating previous legislation and providing the basis for subsequent controls. Some aspects, for example those requiring accurate labelling of the weight and volume of food sold, are more concerned with fair trading than with disease prevention, but the Act also covers such preventive measures as the pasteurization of milk and sets standard upper limits for the addition of preservatives and colouring matters. A series of Diseases of Animals Acts, the first passed in 1894, complement the Food and Drugs Act controlling the production of meat and poultry. Not only food, drink, and drugs are covered by such legislation. The 1961 Consumer Protection Act has led to regulations dealing with the safety of carry-cot stands, fireguards, and other household goods, and the flammability of nightdresses, and the Consumer Safety Bill, which was sponsored by a private member in 1978, will strengthen this type of power. This kind of legislation is also increasingly influenced by the E.E.C. policies (see page 134).

The evolution of legislation

In addition to laws which control individuals' consumption of alcohol and tobacco and those which prevent them being harmed by others, legislation ensures the provision of preventive services. From the Local Government Re-organization Act, which requires local authorities to provide the basic public health services, to those Acts which set up the health and social services, a whole range of legislation requires local and health authorities to ensure the prevention of disease. The enactment of a Bill is only the beginning of the process of social control, however. The new law may be tested and clarified in the courts, it may be amended by a subsequent Act, or it may be adapted and extended by Circulars, Statutory Instruments which must be laid before Parliament for approval, Codes of Practice, and Local Authority Bye-Laws. The enactment of a law is also the end of a process, that of social change. A new law does not come into being solely as the result of the discovery of certain facts: some Acts are passed before the facts of the matter are definitely known, for example the Public Health Act of 1848 (see page 14), and in other cases widely-known and accepted facts do not lead to laws, for example the death and disability which could be prevented by wearing seat belts (see page 79). For a Bill to be introduced there must be political will, and a good deal of luck, as some Bills on prevention have been introduced by the winners of the ballot for Private Members Bills. In the creation of political will many factors operate, among which the pressure groups are increasingly important. The Spastics Society, RoSPA (the Royal Society for the Prevention of Accidents), Age Concern, Help the Aged, the Medical Council on Alcoholism, the British Safety Council, and ASH (Action on Smoking and Health), are only a few of the effective pressure groups. As the mechanism of social change has a certain degree of inertia, however, those groups who wish to oppose legislation are more effective than those who support it. The opponents of fluoridation and the seat belts Bill have been consistently successful although their numbers are small. It is still possible for individuals to exert considerable influence. Sir George Godber when he was Chief Medical Officer to the Department of Health, and David Owen when Minister of State at the Department of Health, were effective from inside the system, and individual campaigners like Michael Daube, formerly Director of ASH, Dr. John Havard, Secretary of the British Medical Association Road Safety Committee, and the backbench M.P.s Sir Bernard Braine and Jack Ashley have shown that the juggernaut momentum of modern central government can be changed.

Education

Messages

Health education has grown steadily more prominent and confident yet the health education movement, like the whole of education, is troubled by two questions: a question of content and a question of style. The content of health education in the 1950s, when the subject was starting to grow, was focused on disease; it was more illness education than health education. The emphasis was on the common causes of death and disability and the means by which they could be prevented. However, health educators became aware that the creation of concern which led to behaviour modification could easily lead to counter-productive anxiety. If too much anxiety is created the educational message is ignored and the person's behaviour is unaltered (see page 145). In the 1970s the emphasis shifted very definitely from illness to health. This was not a new concept; the revolutionary Peckham health centre experiment in the 1930s had 'positive health' as its objective but the scale of the educational effort launched in 1978 was immeasurably greater than any previous attempts. The Health Education Council launched its million pound 'Look After Yourself' campaign with the focus on health promotion rather than illness prevention. The Council asked the rhetorical question 'Why should you bother at all?', and answered

Because it makes you feel good! Life's tough enough already without feeling overweight (bad for ego as well as the heart), tired, tense and hoarse with a smoker's cough. Feeling fit means enjoying life—doing more with the kids, getting in a full weekend before going back to work, looking and feeling more attractive, sleeping better, coping with the problems.

The material offered to the public through television commercials, newspapers, pamphlets, badges, and bookmarks centred mainly on sensible exercise and diet. Whether or not the campaign will achieve its Utopian objective will be extremely difficult to estimate, as its designers must have realized from its inception. It was an act of faith. On a sounder empirical basis was the related 'Living Well' project which was aimed at teenagers. Described as an exercise in 'positive learning' it was similar to the 'positive help' and 'positive activities' of the 'Look After Yourself' campaign and had the same objective of health promotion.

Related to this shift in content was a change in style which took place during the same period, with a trend away from the presentation of information to the presentation of material designed to alter attitudes and value. The informative approach had been effective in some areas. Sir Richard Doll, who had first identified the risk of cigarette smoking with Professor Bradford Hill in their classic study of British doctors, studied the smoking habits of these doctors over two decades and found that the number of cigarettes smoked daily fell from 8.7 in 1951 to 3.6 in 1971 as doctors learned of the dangers of tobacco smoke. The change in smoking habits towards cigarettes with a low tar content owes much to the simple information presented in the Government's 'tar tables', the tar and nicotine yields of the different brands of cigarette as determined by the Government chemist, although it must be said that the industry's pattern of advertising was also influential (see page 163). There was, however, evidence that information alone was insufficient as the smoking habits of hospital nurses demonstrate. Although they have been exposed to a great deal of information, and in spite of the fact that they have seen, met, and nursed people suffering from the diseases caused by smoking, their smoking habits have changed much less than those of doctors.

	General practitioners	Hospital nurses
Percentage currently smoking cigarettes	21	48
Percentage not smoking who used to smoke cigarettes regularly	42	12

Source: *Smoking and Professional People*, Department of Health (H.M.S.O., 1977).

One reason for the failure of education is that it quickly loses its effect. Even the effect of the Government's decision to change the warning on cigarette packets from 'Warning by H.M. Government:

SMOKING CAN DAMAGE YOUR HEALTH' to 'H.M. Government Health Department's WARNING: CIGARETTES CAN SERIOUSLY DAMAGE YOUR HEALTH' in 1977 could have been only short-lived. On the Government tar tables is printed a much more specific warning 'CIGARETTES CAUSE LUNG CANCER, BRONCHITIS, HEART DISEASE' but the tobacco industry opposed the introduction of this warning on packets, as the Employment and Social Services Sub-Committee had recommended, and the Government did not wish to impose this measure because of the benefits they felt they were obtaining from their voluntary agreements with the industry (see page 163). It is probable, however, that neither more frightening information nor more frequent changes of the information presented would increase its effectiveness, and the decision to shift health education away from the informative approach grew from a growing awareness that attitudes and values were as important as knowledge.

The value which a person places on health influences his attitudes towards factors which he knows may affect it, for example someone who values health highly will have a different attitude towards exercise than someone who places a lower value on health. The 'Look After Yourself' and 'Living Well' campaigns were attempts to increase the value people place on health in the hope that this would alter their attitudes towards diet, exercise, and cigarette smoking. The Health Education Council also attempted to influence attitudes directly, without discussing values, by presenting a sexually un-appealing image of people who are cigarette smokers. After a pilot campaign in 1976 the main campaign was introduced in 1978 using the media of commercial advertising. In an advertisement screened in cinemas a girl refuses to kiss her boyfriend, explaining to her friend that 'He's very nice but his breath smells like you'd get lung cancer kissing him'; on a radio commercial a girl says of a boy 'What a let down! His breath reeked of stale tobacco and his mouth tasted like an old fag end.' These were attempts to counter the sophisticated image of smoking. The 'Look After Yourself' campaign also used this approach. Its full page advertisment on obesity was presented under the caption 'Is your body coming between you and the opposite sex?' and the advertisement on exercise had the caption 'You'd enjoy sex more if you had a pair of plimsolls.'

Attempts by governments to influence attitudes and values by means other than the unbiased presentation of facts are more appropriately considered as propaganda than education. Before considering whether or not this approach is ethical, however, it is necessary to consider its effectiveness—whether or not it does influence attitudes and values. Whether the influential approach is more effective, and therefore a more efficient way to spend public money, will take time to evaluate, but research is necessary because the empirical foundations of health education are very weak.

Media

The school is the obvious medium for the health education of children but it is not always easy for the message to be introduced. Although teachers of home economics, biology, and physical education receive some training about health neither they, nor teachers of any other subject, have been taught the range of information necessary to teach health education. This deficiency could be made good by in-service training but neither the Department of Health nor the Department of Education is in a position to organize such training. In the White Paper 'Prevention and Health' these departments expressed the hope that local education authorities would arrange in-service courses on health education for teachers, but stated that this is a decision which each local authority has to make for itself. Furthermore, the Department of Education has no direct control over what is taught in teacher training colleges and many different approaches have developed; some colleges tackle the subject in depth, others are more cursory, but the overall picture is unclear. A research project funded by the Scottish Health Education Unit is currently reviewing the extent of and attitudes towards health education in teacher training colleges, and this should provide information on which a general policy for teacher training can be developed. Scotland is in a fortunate position for it has a Scottish Council for Health Education which is funded by both education authorities and health boards and is probably in a stronger position to develop a comprehensive programme of in-service training than the Department of Education.

Even if this problem were overcome, if teachers were taught the theory of health education, many would find teaching difficult in practice. Education inevitably transmits the attitudes and values prevailing in the culture in which it is set, but in recent years there has been little attempt to impart these didactically through subjects in the curriculum.

Education for personal relationships (E.P.R.) is now taught in some schools, and a growing number of, but not all, teachers are interested in pastoral care. Teachers expect to have to judge what is right on matters of fact, for example whether the tense of a French verb is right, but not every teacher is prepared or able to answer on matters of values, if, for example, a pupil asks whether it is right to have sex before marriage or to smoke cannabis. Even if a teacher feels that he has thought through the issues involved carefully enough to answer he may be hesitant, uncertain whether or not the headmaster, parents, or governors agree with his views and the answer he would give.

Health education faces even greater obstacles in secondary schools because the timetable allows little opportunity for the introduction of new subjects, especially in schools in which preparation for examination receives high priority. One solution would be to make health education an examinable subject at C.S.E., 'O', and 'A' level. Not only would the difficulty of its introduction to timetables which are often already overcrowded still exist but this may not be the best way to educate children about health. Most schools favour an approach which introduces health matters into many subjects, especially biology, home economics (which already includes exam questions on health), physical education (which has a C.S.E. exam including health questions), religious education, and education for personal relationships, with one teacher acting as health education co-ordinator. But even this approach may be too narrow. It is probably insufficient to include health education only in what Basil Bernstein has called the instrumental order of the school, that is its curriculum, and it should also permeate the expressive order of the school, its conduct and culture. Any beneficial effects of teaching pupils about the consequences of smoking in biology lessons are probably nullified if the pupils see teachers smoking in the staff room.

Although the Department of Education has no direct control over school curricula, both the composition and balance being decided by the local education authority, school governors, and the head-master, it exerts a considerable and valuable indirect influence. In

1974 an excellent report on 'Health Education in Schools' was issued to Scottish education authorities and the Department of Education issued a report bearing the same name in 1977. The Schools Council, which is supported by the Department of Education, has played a leading part in developing material for use in both primary and secondary schools, working in collaboration with the Health Education Council and the Scottish Health Education Unit. At local level the key person is the health education officer who is able to advise teachers and ensure that the most appropriate material is available.

Education of adults is more difficult, because there is no single medium through which they can be reached. Use is made of the mass media and public buildings such as libraries and health centres, where posters can be displayed, but this is complementary to the educational efforts of health service professionals, especially health visitors and general practitioners. A health visitor is a State Registered Nurse who has received a further year of training orientated towards the social sciences. Most health visitors work attached to general practice teams and the main emphasis of their work is preventive, whereas the work of district nurses is orientated towards care and cure. Most health visiting is to the homes of mothers with young children but some health visitors are also school nurses, and many spend time with groups of adults, common activities being weight reduction and smoking cessation groups. In 'The Way Forward' the Government's strategic plan for health and social services published in 1977, it was stated that there should be a six per cent annual increase in expenditure on health visiting and district nursing. It is unlikely that this objective will be reached because the training and employment of health visitors is paid for by area health authorities, not by the Department of Health, and many authorities are unable to expand their health visiting service at this rate, even though they may agree in principle with the need for prevention through education, because of the financial constraints within which they have to operate. General practitioners, like many hospital doctors, have become more interested in education as a result of the findings of a number of research projects indicating that as many as fifty per cent of people who had been prescribed drugs were not taking them as the prescribing doctor had intended. Realizing that a doctor had to educate and not merely to instruct patients, the Royal College of General Practitioners developed a training scheme for doctors wishing to enter general practice which includes much more material on education and prevention than an undergraduate medical course contains. As most doctors who wish to become G.P.s now take this training, the interest of general practice in prevention and the skill to educate should steadily increase.

The health education officer also plays an important role in supporting health service staff, in addition to the service he offers to school teachers. Employed by the area health authority and working closely with the area medical officer (in Scotland the chief administrative medical officer) he has to develop a strategy for health education. As their numbers are small, there were fewer than 300 health education officers in Britain in 1977 and their approach has to be mainly indirect. They have to use the local press and radio and work with and through teachers, general practitioners, health visitors, community health councils (in Scotland local health councils), and any other interested individuals or groups to reach as many people as possible. To try to overcome this shortage of health education officers the Department of Health allocated, in both 1977 and 1978, an additional £1 million to the Health Education Council to sponsor the training of its officers, and the Scottish Home and Health Department has subsidized the Scottish Health Education Unit for the same purpose. Both central departments recognized that health authorities and, in Scotland, health boards, were under such financial pressure that they would find it difficult to fund health education, which is an investment with little immediate return, when they were faced with so many pressing demands for extra finance by acute services whose need and benefit was immediately evident (see page 154).

Although it is important to have certain groups of professionals with a special interest in prevention, for example general practitioners, health visitors, and community midwives, it is equally important to involve all health service professionals in prevention. The 'Report of the Committee on Nursing', the Briggs Committee, laid emphasis on the need to educate nurses about preventive medicine and health education, subjects which too often receive little attention at present, and the education of medical students now considers patient education to a much greater degree than hitherto. But much more could still be done to prepare health service professionals for health education.

It is not only health service professionals who are involved in the health education of adults. Environmental health officers are responsible for education on home safety, food hygiene, noise and pollution, and other preventable environmental hazards. The police and road safety training officers, who are appointed by county councils, try to reduce road traffic accidents by the education of cyclists, motor cyclists, and pedestrians, especially those at special risk, for example children and old people. Safety and training officers work with trade union representatives to educate about health and safety at work, receiving advice from the inspectors of the Health and Safety Executive (see page 168). Individual health educators have to be backed by organizations which not only ensure that they receive accurate information for presentation in a style which has been shown to be effective but which also produce pamphlets, posters, and films aimed directly at the public to reinforce the message of the health educators. The Department of Employment supports health education at work, the Home Office is responsible for education about fire hazards, the Department of Prices and Consumer Protection is concerned with home safety, and the Department of Transport with road safety. To approach the public directly these central organizations publish their own information and use the Central Office of Information (C.O.I.), especially for major campaigns. The C.O.I. may produce the necessary material itself or commission an advertising agency, just as though it were a tobacco or drink company. The Department of Health also uses the skills of the C.O.I., but it relies on the Health Education Council for its major educational thrust. The Council and the Scottish Health Education Unit are responsible for the development of health education strategy and for encouraging relevant research. Each has a full-time staff and a board of part-time advisors, appointed by the Secretary of State and drawn from the health and education services, because the Health Education Council has links with schools both directly and through its work with the Schools Council.

It is this involvement of people outside government which is essential if health education is to be successful. Education is not only a matter for government departments and professionals, but must also involve a wide range of organizations and individuals so that it can reach a wide range of people and because some messages will be more effective if they are transmitted in other ways than by government departments or employers. The pressure groups such as RoSPA and ASH obviously have an educational role, but so do many other organizations, for example the Red Cross, St. John Ambulance Association, the Pre-Retirement Association, Help the Aged, and Age Concern.

Although health education receives extensive publicity it is worthwhile to emphasize that its activities are small in comparison with those of advertising. In 1976 about £½ million was spent on education about the dangers of alcohol in comparison with the £36 million spent advertising its pleasures.

Advertising

The change in style of health education from one which was intended to be informative to one which was designed to be influential was motivated by two factors; the realization that attitudes and values influenced decisions, and the appreciation of the growing power of advertising.

Advertising should not be considered in isolation: it is but the end stage of a marketing process by which products are developed on the evidence of market research to meet the wants of the consumer, and only one part of the process of promotion. In 1977 nearly £30 million pounds was spent on the advertising of cigarettes in the cinema, the press, and on hoardings, but the total amount spent on their promotion was in the region of £80 million pounds, sponsoring such sports as football, rugby, and steeplechasing, and subsidizing the arts. The million pounds spent by the Government on health education and smoking is insignificant by comparison. As competition increases, promotion intensifies. In 1978 British American Tobacco, allowed to enter the British market by the Treaty of Rome, introduced State Express 555 in a promotion costing £5 million. Part of this was a £2 million sports sponsorship scheme intended to help sportsmen at all levels, but a similar sum could easily be raised by the government for it amounts to no more than 0.1 per cent of annual government revenue from tobacco. As part of the same promotional 'launch' coupons offering five pence off State Express, already set at an artifically low price to undercut the king-size market, were delivered to 13½ million households.

The expenditure on the promotion of alcohol is of similar magnitude. In 1977 more than £20 million was spent advertising wine and spirits. For example, £3.6 million was spent advertising vermouth in campaigns aimed particularly at young drinkers— Martini alone spent £1.7 million pounds, and the expenditure on advertising rum rose 44 per cent over the 1976 figure. There were, in addition, many other promotions of alcohol. Dewars whisky sponsored a chess championship, Pernod sponsored bowling, Bells awarded money to the football manager of the month, Bass Charrington sponsored squash, Tennant Caledonian sponsored two prom performances of 'The Marriage of Figaro', and William Grant and Sons promoted a Glenfiddich Research Fellowship in Scottish History at St. Andrews University.

What is the influence of advertising? Advertisers claim that it only influences brand loyalty, that is to say it does not stimulate people to start smoking or to increase the amount they smoke. It is true that a ban on the advertising of alcohol in British Columbia did not have a significant effect on the consumption of alcohol and that the consumption of cigarettes and alcohol is high in countries in which there is little advertising, for example in Russia, but there is evidence that advertising does influence the decisions of people to smoke or drink alcohol. Dr. John Treasure, the chairman of the world's largest advertising agency, J. Walter Thomson, said that

There are campaigns in this country which overtly set out to stimulate the total consumption of the product group. It should not, however, be thought that the brand expenditure by a strong market leader does not also have an effect on the size of the total market, even if this is not the overt purpose of the campaign . . .

George Washington Hill, former president of British American Tobacco, who was behind the classic 'reach for a Lucky' campaign, said that 'the impetus of these great advertising campaigns built (success) for ourselves, but built the cigarette business as well, because this is the way competition works.' It seems probable that advertising influences not only brand loyalty, but also the total consumption of alcohol and tobacco.

Learning and the law

Although education and legislation have been discussed separately they are closely interwoven in the prevention of disease.

There is legislation on health education which is, perhaps surprisingly, much more the subject of statute law in America than in Britain. The National Health Planning and Resource Development Act of 1974 directed the Secretary for Health Education and Welfare to develop 'effective methods of educating the general public concerning proper personal health care and effective use of available health services'. The Comprehensive School Education Act and the National Consumer Health Information and Health Promotion Act, both signed by President Ford in 1976, further specified the need for health education. These federal laws are buttressed by state laws. By 1976 sixteen states had passed Acts mandating comprehensive health education programmes, and some states had also passed Acts requiring the inclusion of specific subjects, for example Florida's Drug Abuse Education Act of 1970. There is less central control of school curricula in Britain than in some other countries, but the government is able to influence curricula through the grants it makes available for in-service training of teachers and through the influence of the Health Education Council, the Scottish Health Education Unit, and the Schools Council.

In Britain the law has not been used to specify the content of health education in such detail, merely defining where the responsibility for education lies, for example the National Health Service Reorganization Act 1973 states that 'it shall be the duty of the Secretary of State to provide . . . to such extent as he considers necessary to meet all reasonable requirements . . . facilities for the prevention of illness', a duty delegated both to area health authorities and to the Health Education Council. The Home Safety Act of 1961 defines district councils as having the responsibility for education about hazards in the home and the prevention of home accidents which is implemented by environmental health officers. This brief Act stated that 'a local authority may promote safety in the home by publishing or making arrangements for otherwise giving information and advice relating to the prevention of accidents in the home'. This is permissive legislation, whereas the law on road safety is obligatory. Section 8 of the Road Traffic Act 1974 states that 'each local authority shall prepare and carry out a programme of measures to promote road safety', but does not stipulate educational measures.

A growing body of legislation governs the labelling of products to protect the public. The Packaging and Labelling of Dangerous Substances Regulations 1978 made under the Health and Safety at Work Act (1974) requires suppliers to indicate the properties of substances. The British Standards Institution (B.S.I.) Kitemark signifies that goods such as crash helmets or seatbelts meet certain safety standards and, in 1975, a special B.S.I. electrical safety mark was introduced to complement the British Electro-technical Approvals Board (B.E.A.B.) mark, which is found on approved household electrical appliances. These safety marks are not yet obligatory but the Consumer Safety Bill, a private member's bill introduced in 1978, and the E.E.C. Consumer Protection Act will ensure that this aspect of prevention by education will become increasingly common and important. As legislation plays a larger role in the control of labelling, the range of Government departments involved in education also increases. For example, the Department of Employment controls the labelling of dangerous chemicals, and the Department of Prices and Consumer Protection's role in consumer protection grows steadily as product safety and manufacturers' liability become matters of increasing public concern (see page 175).

Legislation plays a vitally important preventive role in the control of the advertising industry's education service. There is a Code of Advertising Practice supervised by the Advertising Standards Authority which lays down that advertising should be legal, decent, honest, and truthful, but as the A.S.A. is financed by the advertising industry, the Consumer Association and other groups have called for an independent body to supervise advertising. Advertising is, however, coming under increasing control. Cigarette advertising has been banned on commercial television since 1965 and on commercial radio since its inception in 1973. Other advances have been made possible by co-operation with the tobacco industry. The Code of Advertising Practice now stipulates that advertisements should 'not seek . . . to establish that to smoke is . . . associated with a luxurious way of life' and that 'care requires to be

exercised in the use of outdoor settings so as to avoid any implications of health that would be inappropriate being conveyed' and
there are other recommendations precluding the use of heroes of
young people, but the spirit of the Code is not infrequently breached.
To its credit the tobacco industry agreed to spend a dispro-
portionate amount of money on the advertisement of low-tar
cigarettes and to end the advertising of high-tar and middle-to-high
tar cigarettes in 1978, as part of a package of measures agreed with
the Department of Health in 1977. The control of promotion
through sports sponsorship proved more difficult, partly because
of the equivocal attitude of the Minister of Sport. In the White
Paper the Government stated that sports sponsorship was
'inappropriate and unfortunate' but one year later the Minister of
Sport was associated with the State Express 555 £2 million sports
sponsorship scheme.

The State Express promotion evoked a response from the International Athletics Club which placed a half page advertisement in
The Times headed trenchantly 'Get out of Athletics British American
Tobacco', and this type of public action may, in the long run, be
more effective than governmental pressure.

A complete ban on advertising was introduced in Norway in
1975 by the Norwegian Tobacco Act and similarly in Finland in
1978, but such a ban on either cigarette or alcohol advertising
seems unlikely in Britain. The reasons given in the White Paper
were that the evidence that such a ban would be effective was
inconclusive, that the ban 'would be regarded as an unnecessary
restriction on the liberty of the individual', and that it would
counteract the Government's own strategy of using advertising to
encourage people to smoke low-tar brands of cigarette. However, it
did say that it 'would keep an open mind on the question of a total
ban on cigarette advertising'.

There are similar controls on the advertising of alcohol. The
Advertising Standards Authority, the Drink Advertising Working
Party of the Incorporated Society of British Advertisers, and
representatives of the drinks industry produced a special appendix
to the Code of Advertising Practice setting out a number of rules.
For example, it states that advertisements should not 'give the
general impression that drinking is necessary for social success or
acceptance', nor should it 'claim or suggest that any drink can

contribute towards sexual success', but these and other impressions continued to be conveyed by certain advertisements. In advertising, as in many health matters, the emphasis is placed more and more on self-control rather than on external controls. In a remarkable initiative the Distilled Spirits Council of the United States laid plans for $2.5 million of advertising space in influential journals such as *Penthouse* and *Playboy* to promote 'responsible drinking'. This may set a precedent for British advertisers and government to follow. It would seem better to aim for a co-operative approach rather than one which was coercive, because the distinction between state control of advertising for health purposes and censorship is subtle and delicate.

In addition to considering the effect of legislation on education the potential effect of education on legislation should not be forgotten. Mr. Healey has used Budget speeches to emphasize the association between cigarette smoking and disease and to justify his use of taxation as a means of preventive medicine (see page 117) but there have been few other attempts to educate about the role of law, although opportunities exist. Many schoolchildren are now taught civic or social education, and such courses could include material which presents the use of the law as means of prevention in a favourable light. For example, the need for a law to make the wearing of seat-belts compulsory could be presented by emphasizing that those people injured because they were not wearing seat-belts were not only harming themselves but were affecting other people by consuming limited health service resources (see page 157), and the same message could be directed at the public through posters and films.

Education cannot be value-free, but the values are usually transmitted implicitly through the expressive order of the school, its ethos, for example the school's respect for the monarchy or the church; but the introduction of such material to the instrumental order of the school, the curriculum, or to the general public would be controversial. Precedent exists however, and the posters issued by the Ministry of Transport in the period before the introduction of the breathalyser influenced attitudes towards this controversial piece of legislation. Education about legislation is increasingly common but the main educators are not arms of the administration but pressure groups. ASH, RoSPA, and other groups are frequently in the press as they seek to educate the public not only about dangerous substances and practices but about the need for social, fiscal, and legal controls. With a better-educated electorate this aspect of prevention through education will probably grow, but for government itself to try to influence attitudes and values towards proposed legislation by means other than by the straightforward presentation of information probably too closely resembles propaganda for politicians to wish to undertake.

Screening

Although screening is based on legislation and relies on education, it is a means of secondary prevention (see page 33) which requires separate consideration. The concept of screening is deceptively simple. It is based on the fact that, in general, people do not attend their doctors until they have a symptom, and that symptoms may develop some time after the onset of a disease. For example a breast lump is usually noticed after it attains a diameter of several centimetres by which time cancer, if the lump is cancerous, may have progressed to a serious stage. Theoretically, by screening the whole population a disease could be detected at an early, presymptomatic stage and therefore be treated more effectively. On this premise screening gained considerable support in the 1950s and early 1960s. Screening for anaemia, for heart disease, for cervical cancer, and, logically, annual health checks in which individuals were subjected to a whole battery of tests designed to detect a number of diseases became popular.

The concept of screening was not new. The school medical examinations introduced in 1908, regular antenatal examinations, and the developmental assessment of children by health visitors and doctors in infant welfare clinics were well-established procedures, and there were other examples, but the late 1950s and early 1960s saw the rapid, enthusiastic expansion of screening, an expansion which was brought to a halt in the latter half of the 1960s as its problems were recognized. There were practical problems, for example there were not enough medical staff or financial resources to implement all the suggested screening procedures.

There were technical problems such as the realization that the distinction between disease and normality was not clear-cut. For example, medical students had been taught that a certain level of haemoglobin, the oxygen carrying blood pigment, was the lower limit of normal, below which the person was anaemic. Research showed, however, that many people detected by means of screening as having haemoglobin levels below this hypothetical lower limit of normal were not only free from symptoms but were not made to feel any better by treatment with iron tablets. On the contrary some felt worse not only because they were told that they had anaemia but because they were prescribed and consumed iron preparations which had side-effects. There were also reservations on ethical grounds. When an individual with symptoms attends a doctor he expects not only that the doctor will exercise reasonable skill and care in his treatment but also accepts that the relief of his symptom may entail discomfort and danger, even that he may die as the result of an operation. The doctor tries to help the patient obtain relief by the best means he knows, even though success cannot be guaranteed and some risk is entailed. This is implicit in the contract between patient and doctor and is acceptable to both parties. If, on the other hand, a doctor approaches a person who is free from symptoms, examines him, and discovers he has some abnormality, thus creating anxiety, he must be certain that the treatment available for this condition will be effective and free from side-effects. A woman who detects a lump in her breast and fears she has cancer seeks medical help and accepts the need for an anaesthetic and operation as a means to end her fear. If the breast lump is detected on screening, however, it is the doctor who has initiated her fear, anxiety, anaesthetic, and operation. If it transpires that she has cancer, screening can be regarded as justifiable in her case. If, on the other hand, she does not have cancer, is her fear and the risks she has run during anaesthesia and operation justified by the fact that cancer will be found earlier in some other women? Can the unnecessary anxiety and risk of those women who do not have cancer be compared with the benefit which accrues to those who do in a form of utilitarian equation to substantiate the ethical acceptability of screening?

As a result of the recognition of these problems a number of criteria were drawn up against which suggested screening procedures could be assessed to decide whether or not they should be implemented.

- The condition screened for should be an important problem.
- An acceptable test should be available which will diagnose all cases of the disease but which will make falsely positive diagnoses in none of those people who do not have the disease.
- The test should be safe.
- An acceptable, effective treatment and the services necessary to provide it should be available.
- Earlier treatment should give better results than that given at the stage at which symptoms develop.

Certain screening tests survived the test of these criteria. Cervical cytology is now accepted as an effective means of secondary prevention although there is concern that those most at risk, women in social classes IV and V, attend for screening less frequently. Screening for certain uncommon but important congenital causes of mental handicap, such as phenylketonuria (see page 44), and antenatal screening of pregnant women are also of proven value. But under this ethical scrutiny many of the proposed screening schemes were invalidated, in Britain at least. In America, screening, especially the annual health check, persisted for much longer, partly because of the tremendous financial rewards which screening brings when each test and treatment entails a fee.

Others were discontinued because they had become inefficient although they were still effective in the detection of disease. For example, as tuberculosis became less common, mass radiography became inefficient and the detection of new cases by the tracing of contacts of those cases who had presented with symptoms became more appropriate. Special circumstances still necessitate screening for tuberculosis, for example, all teachers are required to have a chest X-ray before starting work with pupils, but this is on a different ethical basis because it is principally for the protection of children.

Other screening procedures have been, or are being introduced, for instance screening for spina bifida (see page 45) and mongolism (see page 44) in pregnancy. Comprehensive screening of old people is not worthwhile but screening aimed at specific problems, for example the need for chiropody, can prevent deterioration in old age (see page 112). Screening for breast cancer is also the subject of debate. The primary prevention of breast cancer being impossible at present, because the cause is unknown, secondary prevention by screening has been tried in several parts of the world. Breast cancer can be detected at an early stage either by mammography, an X-ray of the breast, or by examination by a doctor, or by self-examination, or by a combination of these techniques. Because of this it has been proposed that a national breast screening service with easily accessible clinics be instituted, although the Department of Health has been cautious. In the 1977 White Paper it stated that 'there is not yet sufficient evidence of its effectiveness and efficiency to justify the introduction of a national screening service for breast cancer', and was worried that the exposure of a large number of woment to the radiation of mammography might actually induce cancer in a small proportion of them. However, the Department of Health agreed to set up two trials of the effectiveness of screening. One is to compare the effectiveness of clinical examination, including mammography, with breast self-examination. The other is to study women's attitudes towards screening, and this is of tremendous importance as public participation is essential if screening is to be successful.

7 Obstacles to prevention

Linguistic

Semantic

Preventive medicine has its effect by means of language, for legislation and education are both linguistic media, so its effectiveness is reduced if any of the three components of language—lexical, semantic, or grammatical—are wrongly employed.

The lexical component of language pertains to the words, the vocabulary, used; but this aspect of language now presents only minor problems. Although those who practise prevention have an extensive vocabulary they are careful not to use words like 'myocardial infarction' or 'carcinoma', employing instead the terms 'heart attack' and 'cancer', words which are found in the vocabulary of almost everyone. Careful research is conducted before and after health education material is presented to ensure that the vocabulary used includes only words of common currency.

The semantic component of language pertains to the meaning of the words and terms used. If two people use the same word but each uses it with a different meaning, communication will be blocked. The word 'risk' is frequently used, but it is a word with more than one meaning. To the person interested in preventing disease and death the word implies a situation which has unpleasant connotations which he assumes people will wish to avoid by reducing the risk. For other people, however, the term risk may have different connotations. Young people, especially young males in societies of simple technology, are often intentionally exposed to risk during initiation rites, and risk has therefore connotations of manhood. Although the formal initiation rites in developed societies do not embody risk as an essential element, except the risk of examination failure, risk has a positive utility for many young people in the informal rites of the passage of adolescence. Young people who use the word with such a meaning will not necessarily avoid actions which they are told carry a risk—on the contrary, they may seek them out. The attitude engendered by this meaning of the word risk may be strengthened by the natural and normal tendency of young people to reject advice from parents and other figures of authority as they attempt to define the limits of their own sphere of authority.

The word risk implies probability and this is a universal implication. The likelihood of the occurrence of a probable event can be stated numerically ranging from 0 if the probability is zero, that is if it is certain that the event will not occur, to a probability of 1 for events which are certain to occur. Numerical statements of probability are frequently used in the calculation of the risk of disease but when addressing the public or politicians the probability is stated verbally in adverbs such as 'seldom', 'commonly', 'likely', 'very', 'extremely', 'rather', and adjectives such as 'rare' or 'common', which have different meanings for different people. Research has shown that people are consistent in their ordering of these terms, for example most people rate 'probable' as a statement of greater probability than 'possible', but that there is a range of meanings for each word. For some, a 'probable' event is one which they will seek to avoid; for others, 'probable' implies a risk that can be run.

Neither do the words 'illness' and 'death' have single meanings. To someone trying to promote prevention the word illness implies pain, discomfort, and disability; it implies an unrewarding social condition. To a child, on the other hand, the word illness may connote a rewarding experience which includes extra sympathy, care, and attention, by conferring a status which carries the prerogative of the right to stay off school; it implies a rewarding social condition. Even if the child has experience of a serious illness or injury, which is not common, the memory left with the child who was injured and the image created for other children may still be positive. Consider how rewarding it can be for a child to have a limb in plaster as a result of a road traffic accident. Even though he experiences disability and discomfort he occupies a prominent and privileged position in school which is seen by other children who do not experience the disadvantages. For an adult working in a job which offers little satisfaction the social condition of illness also has its rewarding consequences and therefore the word illness also has a rewarding implication in its meaning (see page 100). To a young person the word 'death' usually has frightening connotations if it relates to a member of his family but when it is used in abstract its impact is much less. To a youngster aged 15 the argument that men who smoke cigarettes sometimes die suddenly at the age of 55 may not have the desired objective to make him stop smoking because the prospect of being 56 years old is not only difficult to imagine but has little appeal. To a 15 year old boy or girl sudden death at 55 is not necessarily as terrible a prospect as it is to the health educator who is nearer the age of 55, although it is highly probable that the prospect of death, sudden or slow, at the age of 55 will seem dreadful to that 15 year old when he or she reaches the age of 54. The fact that a word can have different meanings to the same person at different stages in his life poses particular problems for preventive medicine because the decisions of someone at the age of 15 may affect his health when he is 54.

Grammatical

The linguistic obstacles which stand in the way of preventive medicine are not only lexical and semantic. The linguistic framework, the grammar, in which the words are set can also be a barrier. The grammatical style which is used in prevention is rich in future and conditional tenses, and in the subjunctive mood. For example, 'if you smoke cigarettes it may be that you will suffer heart disease in thirty years' time', is the usual style of argument, but it is a style unfamiliar to many of those people at whom it is aimed. The obstacle is not only grammatical. The two groups are not different simply in their ability to use language; they live in different realities.

Such is our confidence in the reality in which we live that few people question the fact that there is a future which is expressed by the future tense. Einstein shows that the dimension of time in our physical reality is relative, although it can be taken as fixed for the purposes of everyday life, and the work of Benjamin Lee Whorfe highlighted the fact that time as part of our social reality is also relative. Trained as a chemical engineer, Whorfe became a linguist, although he worked as an insurance inspector while doing his research on language, a major part of which was conducted in

Arizona with the Hopi Indians. By an analysis of their language he developed his 'new principle of relativity which holds that all observers are not led by the same physical evidence to the same picture of the universe unless their linguistic backgrounds are similar'. Language creates reality and, as language is the vehicle of culture, there are cultural differences in the realities perceived. The importance of this for preventive medicine centres particularly on the cultural differences in the perception of the future. The Hopi Indians do not have a future tense and there are many other languages which do not have a comparable grammatical structure to the future tense that is taken for granted as a description of reality in Indo European languages. Those cultures which are related to agrarian economies have a future which is limited by the annual cycle of seasons on which their life is based. There may be a few long-term plans, for example saving for a daughter's dowry, but the concept of the future is poorly developed. This is not only a feature of underdeveloped countries. In industrialized nations long-term planning is becoming steadily more dominant at a strategic level but at a personal level the concept of the future is frequently curtailed by the process of industrialization which cuts workers off from their rural, annual time-cycle and introduces them to a weekly time-cycle. Those who are employed weekly and rent their house week-by-week live in a very different temporal reality from those people living in mortgaged houses who have insurance policies stretching three or four decades ahead, and who work in secure, superannuated jobs. The practitioners of preventive medicine mostly experience a social and temporal reality which stretches decades into the future, while those at whom their messages are principally directed, because they have higher mobility and mortality rates (see page 152), experience a reality in which the future finishes next Friday. It is true that legislation has made both house and job more secure, reducing the likelihood that either can be lost at short notice, and that insurance cover now extends much more widely, but the effects of this increased security will take time to affect culture, language, and reality. It is important not to think that all the people who live in such economic insecurity belong to a unitary 'culture of poverty' but there is an immediacy about working-class life which influences the way in which the propositions of preventive medicine are interpreted.

What is proposed is usually an immediate course of action while what is promised is usually a benefit, often only the probability of benefit (see page 153), in a future that is twenty or thirty years away. The new style of health education advertisements which attempt to influence attitudes (see page 125) also offer a more immediate reward to young people who stop smoking. This immediate approach is particularly important when trying to convince young people: children who come from a mortgaged, superannuated, insured culture are more likely to adopt their parents' views of the future during socialization than those brought up in a more immediate culture, for example a higher proportion of the former group postpone leaving school, but even they have a poorly developed concept of the future. Preventive medicine must take greater account of the cultural diversity and therefore the diverse realities which co-exist in an apparently unitary culture such as Britain.

Psychological

Defences against anxiety

Perhaps because so many people are now prescribed tranquillizing drugs, anxiety is widely regarded as a dysfunctional condition, a disease. Anxiety can be disabling but it is also a component of normal functioning and plays an essential role in prevention; anxiety can be constructive as well as destructive. It is anxiety which stimulates a mother to protect her child by immunization, which reminds a child to look for traffic before crossing the road, and which influences an adult to decide to stop smoking.

   Decisions are not only made on the basis of information. They involve both cognitive and emotional factors and the aim of health education is not only to inform but to influence the reaction evoked by the information to create productive anxiety (see page 125). Someone is told about the dangers of smoking, becomes anxious, decides to stop, and stops, thus relieving his anxiety. If, however, he is told and accepts that smoking increases the probability that he will develop cancer and heart disease but is unable to stop smoking he has to use defensive techniques to reduce his inevitable anxiety to a tolerable level. Anxiety which cannot be effectively resolved can also be created if someone is bombarded with too many health education messages. If he is informed that smoking, and obesity, and lack of exercise, and drinking before driving, and a number of other activities which are part of his everyday life endanger it, more anxiety is created than he can manage by taking the necessary actions which would require him to change his life-style completely. He, too, has to raise defences against anxiety and these defences are obstacles to prevention.

Various defences are employed. A smoker who cannot stop may reduce his anxiety by citing someone who engages in the risk behaviour safely, for example a relative who has smoked for sixty years; he may adopt a fatalistic approach like the 'bullet with my number on it' defensive technique used by soldiers; he may cite one piece of evidence which posits that smoking is not harmful; or he may develop a ritual which gives him the illusion that he has his smoking under control, for example never smoking in the afternoon. These are ineffective techniques for stopping smoking but they are effective techniques for reducing anxiety. Similar techniques are used to allay anxiety about driving, especially after drinking, and all other activities which are known to carry a risk. Such statements are sometimes called 'irrational' or 'illogical' by those trying to educate but this presupposes that an individual has only one objective in life, namely the reduction of the risk of illness to as low a level as possible. Most people have this objective but they have others too, one of which is the reduction of anxiety to as low a level as possible. If an individual cannot reduce his risk of illness and therefore his anxiety by stopping smoking then he may choose to reduce his anxiety by use of a defence mechanism. To use such a technique is both rational and logical, although it does not reduce the risk of illness. 'The employment of ineffective techniques to allay anxiety when effective ones are not available' is classified as magic by Keith Thomas in his seminal book on the ways in which people manage the anxiety created by uncertainty, *Religion and the Decline of Magic*. Science and magic are not mutually exclusive; many individuals use both every day (see page 17). People use scientific methods such as the analysis of causality to solve problems causing anxiety but if a problem cannot be resolved science is suspended and the individual uses magic to allay the anxiety. The employment of magic to allay anxiety will almost certainly increase because a number of trends make it probable that the level of anxiety in society will increase in many individuals.

Research will reveal the causes of more diseases and each time a cause is revealed anxiety is created among those who wish to avoid the disease, with even greater anxiety among those who are made aware that they are already at risk. If, for example, it is established that the probability of cancer of the cervix is related to the number of sexual partners a woman has had, which is suggested by recent research, anxiety will be created each time sexual intercourse with a new partner is considered and those who have had sexual intercourse with a number of partners will be anxious on that account.

Anxiety will also be increased by the changing nature of the relationship between patients and doctors. Paradoxically, the more effective medicine becomes the less confidence patients have in doctors, or doctors in themselves. Seventy years ago the laity had confidence in doctors who had few effective treatments to offer. Nowadays many criticisms are voiced of doctors who have a whole armamentarium of effective treatments at their disposal. The key to this paradox is that medicine has only become more effective because it has become less certain. It is only because doctors admitted to themselves and to their patients that they were uncertain of the effects of their intervention that ineffective treatments were discovered and weeded out. Uncertainty is the basis of science and scientific medicine is full of it, but this uncertainty contributes to the creation of anxiety. The confident diagnoses and elaborate treatments of the past were not effective means of cure but they were effective means of reducing anxiety. Doctors used magic to relieve the anxiety of their patients and themselves but they are now less willing to do this. Although doctors are being better trained in the reduction of anxiety by means other than tranquillizing drugs or magic, for example by being open and honest with a dying patient, the uncertainty of the honest approach of modern scientific medicine will not allay anxiety about illness and death as much as the magical approach of the past.

The management of anxiety about illness has to be considered in the context of the other anxieties which affect modern society. The fast-changing pluralistic systems of values make decision-making increasingly difficult; the secularization of society removes an effective means of allaying anxiety from a growing proportion of the population (see page 95), and the increasing dangers of life in an industrialized nuclear age all contribute to the growth of anxiety and necessitate the development of magical techniques or the use of anaesthetic drugs such as alcohol to reduce it to bearable levels. Anxiety about illness may appear more manageable than anxiety about nuclear war or some other external threat because effective means of allaying the anxiety are within the individual's power to control, but the very fact that an individual has charge over the cause of anxiety, for example his smoking or over-eating, often increases it. Many people can carry the anxiety created by nuclear missiles because they feel free from any decisions which affect the probability of their use whereas they are intimately involved with decisions governing their smoking and eating habits.

An appreciation of the importance of anxiety is growing, albeit slowly. The British Safety Council and the Tavistock Institute conducted research on the social and psychological aspects of road safety, and research workers at the Christie Hospital in Manchester have shown that a higher proportion of women will attend for cervical cytology if their anxiety that cancer is incurable is first recognized and overcome. Decisions about a risk are made only after it is recognized and man's natural defences against anxiety are often an obstacle to the conscious recognition of risk.

The willingness to gamble

Assuming that an individual comprehends the linguistic information given him about a hazard to his health, and that he is able to manage the anxiety such information creates sufficiently to contemplate its probability, his decision whether or not to act in the way suggested to reduce the risk is determined by risk-benefit analysis. He weighs the benefits of the risk against the magnitude of the consequence of the risk and the probability that it may occur. For example he has to compare the social, psychological, and physical pleasures of smoking with its possible consequences and the probability that any of them may affect him. Risk-benefit analysis is a very widely-used technique. Gambling and insurance are two human activities in which this type of analysis is used by people of many different cultures and levels of intelligence and research in these fields has produced results of relevance to preventive medicine.

It has been found that the decision to take risk is often influenced more by probability than by the consequence. Many people are

more inclined to run a risk of low probability even if the consequence is dire than a risk of high probability of less consequence.
For example, although the consequence of not wearing a seat-belt
can be very severe, the probability of death occurring is so low that
many people are prepared to run the risk. It has been calculated
that the probability of being killed in a road traffic accident in 50
years of driving, about 40,000 trips, is no more than 100 to 1.
People do gamble on football pools in which the possible rewards
are high and the probability of success is low, but the treble-chance
is not a typical form of risk-benefit analysis because the gambler
receives so many other benefits; the chance to exercise skill; the
rituals of coupon filling and checking, and, perhaps the greatest
benefit, the opportunity to dream about his future 'when I win the
pools'.

Research on the purchase of insurance by people living in the
Mississippi flood plain, which is subject to severe destruction at
very irregular intervals several times a century, supports the
contention that people are more influenced by probability than by
pay off, many being unwilling to insure against flood. The insurance
industry's dictum that 'insurance is never bought—it's always
sold' exemplifies their approach which has similarities to some
aspects of preventive medicine. In both, the individual is exhorted
to engage regularly in behaviour which is contrary to his primary
impulses for no more than the promise of a probable pay off in a
distant future. People are so reluctant to behave in this way that
rules have been made to compel them, for example the building
societies' requirement of insurance cover on the life of the person
paying a mortgage and compulsory National Insurance contributions, but the insurance industry, like preventive medicine,
relies on persuasion as well as compulsion. Studies of insurance
buying suggest that health educators could present the risks of
illness more effectively by using the techniques of the insurance
salesmen. It has been found that people over-estimate the probability of improbable events, for example death by lightning, and
under-estimate the probability of common causes of death, for
example death due to cigarette smoking. More information on the
relative probabilities of different hazards could perhaps influence
decision-making. Attitudes can also be influenced by the way in
which the risk is presented. Risks should be presented as prob-

abilities. Preventive medicine is impressed by the fact that 50,000 deaths are caused by cigarettes every year whereas an individual who smoked would probably be more influenced if he were told that the odds that he might become ill were 10 to 1 or less, as the case might be. Attitudes to risk can be influenced by using figures which show lower probabilities. Paul Slovic, an American research worker, suggested that advice on road accident prevention should use figures based on the probability of disabling injury rather than death, because the former is forty times more common. The figures can also be made more effective and the argument more persuasive by expressing the risk over a longer time-span. For instance, instead of stating that the probability of a fatal accident occurring to someone who drives 15,000 km per year is 2,000 to 1 per annum, it can be expressed as being 50 to 1 over a 40 year span.

It is not only individuals who take risks. Society, or at least its elected representatives, take risks. Politicians rarely consider clear-cut issues, although debates are often polarized by the bipartisan nature of British politics. They have to consider not only the econometrician's evidence, which is statements of probability, but also what is practicable. They often have to decide on an acceptable level of risk. For example, many of the preservatives and colouring matter used in food cannot be said to have been definitely proved to be safe for human consumption, yet the Government and the public accepts that they can be regarded as being safe for practical purposes, provided that their concentration is kept below certain levels. The 'Preservatives In Food Regulations' and the 'Colouring Matter In Food Regulations', both made under the Food and Drugs Act 1955, prescribe concentrations which must not be exceeded, for example there must be not more than 70 milligrams of ethyl−4−hydroxybenzoate per kilo of beer. Such definite rules do not delineate safe from unsafe. Similarly, the maximum permissible levels of chemicals allowed in the atmosphere, earth, or water are arbitrary levels, chosen with respect to both the practicability and the cost of control. Political decision-making is influenced not only by considerations of probability, ethics (see page 156), and practicability: other factors are influential, notably emotion. Certain risks to health evoke a greater emotive response than others. Debates on the risks of nuclear power stations are conducted in a different manner to those on the safety of the motor car, not only because radioactive material is a greater potential hazard but because of the demonology which surrounds radio-activity. Emotion also influences individual decision-making. The manner in which an individual evaluates a risk that affects his life is quite different from the manner in which he evaluates a risk to the life of his child. Emotion heightens the anxiety which the uncertainty of risky situations invariably causes.

Empirical

During the last hundred years many of the factors which cause disease have been discovered. Bacteriology in the nineteenth century and epidemiology (see page 29) in the twentieth century laid reliable empirical foundations for prevention, yet ignorance is still a major obstacle to prevention. In some areas ignorance is complete. Sir Richard Doll has suggested that 90 per cent of cancers are environmental in origin but the causes of fewer than half are known for certain; although there are some exciting clues, the cause of multiple sclerosis is still a mystery; in spite of the fact that a great deal is understood about rheumatoid arthritis its primary cause is unknown, and there are many other diseases in which complete ignorance precludes prevention.

There are some diseases the causes of which have been identified but without sufficient accuracy to provide a basis for effective prevention. For example, a number of factors are known to be associated with the increasing frequency of alcohol abuse but the very number of factors involved is a source of confusion to those who wish to prevent this problem. Sometimes different authorities hold differing and conflicting views. Nutrition is one area in which there is confusion and conflict. Most nutritionists now believe that the intake of fats is the most important factor to prevent heart disease, but some of them believe that it is the particular type of fat consumed which is important, whilst others maintain that it is the consumption of purified carbohydrate, sugar, which matters most, and still others, for example the McCarrison Society, that a deficiency in the fibre content of the diet is what should be emphasized most strongly. The food policies which should be developed and the educational messages which should be promoted obviously have to balance these different opinions but where the balance should be struck is itself a matter of opinion, and this uncertainty vitiates the preventive effort. Although the report on the Prevention of Coronary Heart Disease put forward firm recommendations for a prudent preventive diet (see page 64), the Government White Paper on Prevention and Health was much more cautious, stating that 'it is far from easy for the Government to produce clear, straightforward advice applicable to the public generally'. The prevention of mental illness is in an even more confused state. Not only have many possible causal factors been identified and not only are there conflicting opinions as to the relative importance of these theories, but the nature of the phenomenon which is called mental illness is uncertain. For example, some say it is a biochemical illness, others a symptom of a sick society (see page 93). This confusion precludes prevention.

The greater the number of possible causal factors, the more difficult the evaluation of their relative importance. Two of the greatest challenges to prevention in Britain are the social class and regional differences in mortality and morbidity and these exemplify this principle. The difference in the death and disease rates in different social classes is striking and shocking. Almost every cause of death and disease is more common in social classes IV and V (partly skilled and unskilled) than in social class I and II (professional and managerial), even peptic ulceration and coronary heart disease which are usually considered 'executive diseases'.

Standardized mortality ratios of males aged 15–64 years for selected causes of death, England and Wales, 1961 (All classes = 100).

| Cause of death | Social class | | | | |
	I Profes-sional	II Inter-mediate	III Skilled	IV Partly Skilled	V Unskilled
All causes	76	81	100	103	143
Tuberculosis	40	54	96	108	185
Cancer of lung	53	72	107	104	148
Coronary disease	98	95	106	96	112
Bronchitis	28	50	97	116	194
Ulcer of duodenum	48	75	96	107	173

Source: *Prevention and Health: Everybody's Business* (H.M.S.O., 1976).

The same trend shows for still births and infant mortality (see page 56). The regional differences are less dramatic but are still a cause for concern. If a line can be drawn from the Wash to the Bristol Channel those people living north of the line have, on average, a shorter life span, higher mortality rates at all ages, and higher disease rates than those south of the line. For example, the standardized mortality ratio (see page 75) for the Newcastle Regional Hospital Board was 112 in 1972 (national standardized mortality ratio = 100); in the Oxford region it was 87. In 1975 the infant life wastage, the number of stillbirths and deaths under one year of age, ranged from 32.7 per thousand births in the west of Scotland to 23.1 per thousand in East Anglia. Many factors can be identified which could contribute to regional and social class differences and the two problems overlap, for, if London which has special health problems is excluded, the south east of Britain has proportionately less people in social classes IV and V than the north and west. Whether the important factors are the higher smoking rates, or poverty, or diet, or air pollution, or the effect of the different working conditions, or whether they are genetic, influenced by the migration of people from the north and west, is undecided, and this indecision hinders prevention. The Department of Health has set up research projects to try to determine the answers but they will not be easy to identify.

Finally, knowledge about the causes of disease is obtained by studying groups of people and applying statistical techniques but the knowledge gained in this way is difficult to apply directly to an individual. For example, although it is certain that life-expectancy decreases as obesity increases not all obese people die prematurely so it is difficult to know how strongly to advise or exhort an overweight individual to lose weight because our knowledge of all the factors involved is incomplete. The White Paper was cautious on giving advice on diet, not only because the evidence was incomplete, but because 'individuals' metabolism, and material circumstances vary'.

Many organizations are involved in research. The Medical Research Council, the Social Science Research Council (now involved in smoking research), the Health Education Council, the Scottish Health Education Unit, Regional and Area Health Authorities, central government departments, the British Safety

Council, the Royal Society for the Prevention of Accidents, and the Consumers' Association are some of the principle sources of research initiative. Research has two main emphases, to uncover causes and, an increasing area of interest, to uncover reasons why individuals do not act on the information they are given. Research on the causes requires basic scientific and epidemiological skills (see page 27). Different skills—anthropological, sociological, psychoanalytic, historical, and psychological—are required to investigate the linguistic and psychological obstacles and provide a more secure empirical framework for effective prevention.

Financial

The law which made the wearing of crash helmets compulsory cost little to implement in financial terms, but preventive medicine is not always so cheap. In underdeveloped countries cost is frequently an obstacle to prevention, as has already been discussed (see page 39), but cost can also stand in the way of progress in developed countries.

The cost of prevention must be considered in terms of the benefits which it is thought will ensue if these measures are implemented before the true cost can be calculated. The cost of screening for and preventing spina bifida (see page 45), for example, has to be compared not only with the health service costs of treating children born with this condition but also with the cost of special education, housing, social services, social security payments, and the potential loss of productivity of disabled people. Consideration should also be given to the emotional problems of the disabled people and those who support them, particularly their families. Set in these terms the expense of prevention can be regarded not as a cost but as an investment. Unfortunately, the returns from investment in prevention often take several years to accrue to an amount equal to the cost of prevention. This, together with the fact that it is very difficult to transfer the savings made in education and other services to the obstetric department which has to provide the preventive service, has meant that screening for spina bifida cannot be funded by the diversion of saved resources. Because resources could not be re-allocated to pay for screening, area health authorities had to fund it as a new service and, as it was introduced at a time when there was very little money available for expansion, the service was very slow to develop in some parts of the country. Realizing that preventive services offering the public deferred benefits will always have difficulty in winning resources in competition with hard pressed curative services which offer immediate benefits, it has been suggested that the Department of Health should provide special resources for prevention.

The cost-benefit analysis is more complicated in the case of cigarette smoking. The costs of cigarette smoking—the utilization of health services, the payment of sickness benefit and widows' benefits, and the cost to industrial productivity—have to be set against the financial 'benefits', the retirement pensions 'saved' because smokers die prematurely. Any reduction in cigarette smoking not only alters this balance but it reduces the revenue from tobacco taxation, £1,679 million in 1976, which helps to fund all these services. However, the product of successful prevention is not a commodity like stainless steel which can be accurately valued, it is human life and the techniques of cost-benefit analysis have their limitations when the invaluable is being considered.

The value of a human life can be calculated in a number of different ways; by the value of production lost by death or disability at a certain age, by the amount of insurance an individual is prepared to take out, or, most useful for preventive medicine, by the amount of money society is prepared to spend to save a life. This can be determined by examining policy decisions which have been taken, or not taken, to save life and calculating the costs of these decisions per life saved. Thus the costs of a certain preventive measures have to be compared not only with the benefits of prevention but also with the other preventive measures which could be implemented with those resources. As resources are scarcer than the opportunities for prevention society must consider its priorities for prevention and, even more important, the method by which these priorities are to be decided.

Values of life inferred from several public policy decisions

Decision	Implied value of life	Comment and source
Not to introduce child-proof drug containers	£1,000 maximum	In 1971 the Government decided not to proceed with the child-proofing of drug containers.
Legislation on tractor cabs	£100,000 minimum	In 1969 the fitting of cabs to farm tractors, to reduce mortality risk for drivers, was made compulsory. The cost per annum was estimated at £4m. (£40 for each of 100,000 tractors). About 40 lives would be saved yearly.
Changes in building regulations as a result of partial collapse of Ronan Point high-rise flats	£20,000,000 minimum or perhaps actual	After a high-rise block of flats partially collapsed, killing some residents, the report of the inquiry recommended changes in the building standards of such blocks. It has been estimated from the change in risk and the costs involved that the implied value of life was £20m.
Not to provide treatment for chronic renal failure for a person aged 50	£30,000 (O.H.E. estimate 1976/77 prices)	Particularly in regions where facilities are in short supply, a person over the age of 45 or 50 may stand little chance of being accepted for treatment by dialysis or transplantation.

Source: *Renal Failure* Office of Health Economics (H.M.S.O., 1978).

Ethical

Medical ethics debates usually focus on abortion, euthanasia, and similar clinical topics but preventive medicine also bristles with ethical dilemmas. The topics discussed so far, even the section on the use of legislation in prevention (see page 115), have covered what is possible—what *can* be done. A growing field of concern is what *ought* to be done—on what ethical principle is preventive medicine based? A person with a symptom who attends a doctor expects that the doctor will treat him confidentially with reasonable skill and care, within the constraints set by the facilities he has at his disposal. The basic principle is reasonably clear, but what principle underlies the intervention of the state by legislation, screening, and education in the life of symptom-free, unworried individuals, to prevent them developing, or, to be more accurate, decreasing the probability that they may develop a disease? The contract between doctor and patient is very different from that between citizen and state.

One of the foundations of British Jurisprudence is the essay by John Stuart Mill 'On Liberty'. Written in 1859 its theme is encapsulated in his famous statement that

the only purpose for which power can rightfully be exercised over any member of a civilized society is to prevent harm to others. His own good, either physical or moral, is not a sufficient warrant. He cannot rightfully be compelled to do or forbear because it will be better for him to do so or because it will make him happier, or because in the opinion of others to do so would be wise or even right. These are good reasons for remonstrating with him, or reasoning with him, or persuading him or entreating him, but not for compelling him.

On this definition the Public Health Act, which protects individuals from harm by third parties is ethically acceptable, whereas a law which would make the wearing of seat-belts compulsory would not be. It could be argued that J. S. Mill's statement has been invalidated as a criterion by changing economic circumstances. In 1859 a person who became ill was mainly a burden on his family. Today a person who becomes ill and uses the health service affects other people, for the resources he uses cannot be given to them. In 1859 only one-tenth of the national income was spent on public services. J. S. Mill might have had a very different opinion had he lived in a society in which one-half of the national income was expended by the State for the good of the individual citizens. His attitude would probably also have differed had he known that more than one-tenth of that public expenditure was spent on a finite health service faced by more needs than it can satisfy. Anyone who becomes ill by his own actions affects the services received by other people and may therefore affect their freedom. Someone severely injured in a car crash because he was not wearing a seat-belt may cost the health service £1,000, which means £1,000 less to spend on renal transplantation, chiropody, or any other of the services which are at present inadequate.

Public and political attitudes towards suggested government actions to reduce the probability of disease and death are influenced by considerations other than J. S. Mill's criterion. Many treatments which are not of conclusively proven effectiveness are given to people who seek relief of symptoms, providing that no more effective treatment is available. However, because of the contract between citizen and state on which preventive medicine is based, a much greater degree of certainty has to be attained before measures can be suggested.

Even if certain that a course of action will prevent disease the possibilities that it might be harmful to some people raises ethical obstacles, no matter how many more people will benefit than will suffer. One of the arguments used against the seat-belt Bill was that some people would be killed or injured in accidents because they were wearing seat belts which they would not have worn had there been no law, although it was conceded by opponents of the Bill that the number injured or killed would be very much less than the number who would be saved.

The ethical acceptability of proposed legislation depends also on the nature of the sanction intended. There was some political opposition to the use of taxation to raise cigarette prices and reduce consumption but the public has accepted that the use of taxation for this objective is right, although not every member of the public realises that this is one of the reasons for price increases, even if they do not welcome it. In contrast, the suggestion that random breath-testing should be introduced has been vehemently resisted both because of the nature of the sanction applied to criminal offences and because it extended the powers of the police.

Even if the sanction of a proposed law is acceptable its enforcability influences attitudes towards its introduction. There is a feeling that the State ought not to introduce the legislation on seat-belts because, being difficult to enforce, it would be neither obeyed nor respected and would contribute to a loss of respect of the law in general.

Often more than one consideration is pertinent. The law which makes the possession or smoking of cannabis an offence is attacked not only because it breaches J. S. Mill's fundamental principle but also because it makes these acts criminal offences and its enforcement is difficult. Some people who smoke cannabis not only have lost respect for that law but for the law in general as a result of their treatment by the police and the law. Those who wish to see cannabis legalized also argue that it is, on present evidence, less harmful to individuals and to society than either alcohol or tobacco. Although the evidence on the effects of cannabis is still incomplete it seems sensible to try to dissuade people from the ingestion of cannabis, or any other unnecessary chemical, but the use of legislation which a substantial number of people consider unethical has serious ethical side-effects. Prohibition remains a signal warning on the inappropriate use of legislation.

It has been suggested that ethical problems can be solved linguistically. For example, in its White Paper, the Government stated that 'before it could support a policy of outright banning of cigarette advertising the merits of doing so would need to be confirmed beyond doubt'. By inverting this sentence it could be proposed that cigarette promotions should be banned outright unless the tobacco industry can prove beyond doubt that advertising does no harm, but this is not the same proposition. The proposition posited in the White Paper gives the advantage to citizens, albeit only a group of them, the tobacco industry, and not to the State; the latter gives the advantage to the State. This is the central ethical issue: what should be the balance between the rights of the individual citizens and the imperatives of society?; what part should the law play in bringing about the balance?; and how should these decisions be reached? There is no unanimous opinion. Some jurists maintain that the law should be simply a set of rules based on Millian principles to prevent individuals from harm by others, while it is argued by other jurists that the law should express and enforce moral principles, for example by the proscription of homosexuality between consenting adults, in a more paternalistic role, which would embrace legislation to prevent self-destruction. An opinion which is, however, widely held, is that whatever the role of law there can be too much of it and that a surfeit of legislation has undesirable effects. How much law is too much law? That also is a matter of opinion, another ethical judgement. The Conservative Party would set the limit lower than the Labour Party, and Britain probably uses legislation as a means of preventing disease less than other European countries. The individual wishes freedom from disease, but he also wishes freedom from excessive State intervention.

8 Prevention in practice

Cigarette smoking

The best that can be claimed for the attempts to prevent the abuse of alcohol is that they are slowing down the rate at which the problems are increasing. With cigarette smoking prevention has been more successful. The proportion of men who smoke cigarettes, and the total amount of cigarette tobacco smoked has decreased, most markedly since 1973.

There are a number of other encouraging trends: in 1960 only sixteen per cent of cigarettes smoked were filter-tipped, in 1977 nine out of ten cigarettes were tipped; in 1965 the average tar yield per cigarette was 30 mgm., in 1977 the average tar yield was 17½ mgm. Although it is not yet certain precisely how cigarettes cause disease, the reduction in the consumption of tar resulting from the change to filter tips and cigarettes with a lower tar and nicotine yield reduces the harmful effects of cigarette smoking. There are other trends which are less encouraging, particularly the fact that some people are increasing their cigarette consumption. About 50,000 people still die each year from cigarette smoking, principally because of lung cancer, heart disease, and bronchitis. The lung cancer rate is certainly decreasing in men (see page 69) but the same disease is increasing in women, reflecting their accelerating cigarette consumption (see figure below). This is alarming, as is the increasing difference between the social classes.

Percentage of people smoking, Great Britain

Social class	Men		Women	
	1958	1975	1958	1975
I and II	56	36	43	33
III	60	48	42	45
IV and V	57	52	42	45

Source: *Smoking and Professional People*, Department of Health (H.M.S.O., 1977).

Prevalence of smoking

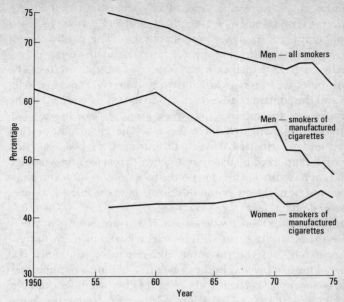

Source: *Prevention and Health*, Cmnd. 7547 (H.M.S.O., 1977).

UK Sales of Tobacco as Cigarettes

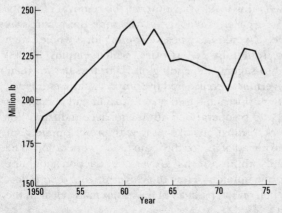

Source: Tobacco Research Council in *Prevention and Health*, Cmnd. 7547 (H.M.S.O., 1977).

A number of factors have contributed to the decline. Education has had an effect. The Royal College of Physicians has issued three major reports on smoking, in 1962, 1971, and 1977, which received wide publicity and influenced public opinion. The publication of the 'league tables' setting out the different tar and nicotine yields of cigarettes in 1973 helped in the switch to low-tar cigarettes. The prohibition of cigarette advertising on commercial radio and television and the control of advertising contributed by weakening the effectiveness of the tobacco industry's attempts to educate. The increasingly sophisticated advertising of the Health Education Council and the Scottish Health Education Unit has also been influential, reinforced by teachers and health service professionals. Legislation has also had an effect—the most important factor since 1973 having been the government's decision to use fiscal measures to control demand (see page 117).

The White Paper on *Prevention and Health* proposed a strategy based on these basic plans with a welcome commitment to fund more research, but the proposals did not meet with universal support. Those interested in the prevention of illness thought they did not go far enough. The Royal College of Physicians, for example, had proposed in its 1977 report *Smoking or Health* the withdrawal of all cigarettes yielding more than 15 mgm. of tar, or 1 mgm. of nicotine—the relative importance of tar, nicotine, and carbon monoxide, which is also produced when tobacco burns, are as yet unknown. As this would have meant the removal of eighty per cent of all the cigarettes smoked at the time the report was compiled, the effects would have been crippling for a whole range of organizations from tobacco factories, which employ 30,000 people, to small newsagents depending on cigarette sales for their survival. The Government considered the proposal 'far too drastic', preferring a gentler approach based on 'education and persuasion of the individual and co-operation with the tobacco industry. For persuasion to work, it must be in keeping with public opinion but generally one step ahead of it. For the industry's co-operation to be secured it is equally important that Government action should be seen to reflect public opinion'. How the Government could reflect public opinion when one step ahead of it was not made clear in the White Paper.

Others felt that the Government had gone too far, opposing their proposals on both practical and ethical grounds, and their opposition was hardened by the Chancellor's decision to introduce a special tax on cigarettes with a tar yield of more than 20 mgm. per cigarette in the 1978 Budget. The industry claimed that such a tax was impractical (because 20 mgm. falls in the middle of the Government's 'Middle Tar' group of cigarettes), unethical (see page 158), and, worst of all, that it broke the spirit of the agreement worked out by industry and Government in 1977, which had included such measures as a voluntary agreement to stop advertising cigarettes in the 'high' and 'middle to high' tar groups (see page 135), the gradual reduction of the tar content of all cigarettes, and the phasing out of cigarettes in the 'middle to high' and 'high' tar groups. The industry had also agreed to try to encourage the trend to low-tar cigarettes by its advertising and pricing policy (see page 172).

A policy based on the proposed measures will persuade an increasing number of people to make the decision to stop smoking. The ways and means of making people decide to stop are known, but it is still uncertain how to help those to have made the decision actually to stop, and how to dissuade young people from starting. Surveys have found that more than two-thirds of smokers wish to stop but of those who try only 25 per cent are successful, no matter what method is used; and many techniques are in current use, for example individual counselling by a G.P., the use of smoking cessation aids, and self-help groups. People are dependent both on the chemicals in tobacco smoke and on the social and psychological benefits of smoking, such as the offer of a cigarette to help establish a relationship or the use of a cigarette to occupy one's hands in a social situation in which one is ill at ease. A better understanding of the physical, social, and psychological factors is necessary if a higher proportion of those who decide to stop can be helped to do so. Young people start to smoke because they want to fulfil certain social needs, such as the wish to appear grown-up. Unfortunately, many who start for such reasons find themselves unable to stop. Sound research has been conducted on the smoking habits of children and young people but an effective educational approach has not yet been developed.

Finally, it seems certain that the rights of the non-smoker will be increasingly respected. There is some evidence that smoke inhaled passively from the cigarettes of other people causes illness and could be regarded as a nuisance (see page 16). Smoke-free zones in public places are becoming more common as non-smokers become more assertive. By the end of this century cigarette smoking may be a comparatively minor problem in Britain, but, as ASH, and War on Want made clear in a report *Tomorrow's Epidemic: Tobacco and the Third World*, published in 1978, it will be a major problem in developing countries as the tobacco companies turn their attention towards these uncontrolled markets.

Alcohol

Specific preventive measures may be directed at the acute problems caused by alcohol abuse, for example drinking and driving, but as these problems often occur in a context of chronic alcohol problems the prevention of such acute problems requires the prevention of chronic excessive consumption (see page 110). One approach would be to identify those drinkers who are more at risk of developing chronic drink problems and concentrate on them, but as this is difficult to do with confidence, a preventive strategy has been developed which has the objective of reducing the total consumption of alcohol, on the premise that the number of people with serious drink problems in any society is in proportion to the total amount of alcohol consumed by the whole society. To this end the Secretaries of State for Social Services, and for Wales, appointed an Advisory Committee on Alcoholism in 1975 and the first report of its sub-committee on prevention, published in 1977, suggested a strategy which embraced the use of both education and legislation. The sub-committee rejected a draconian approach but recommended that none of the existing legal provisions should be relaxed, for example recommending that licensing hours should not be extended, and that some laws should be more rigorously enforced, particularly those applying to young people. The suggestion was made that magistrates should consider the social desirability of applications for new licences, especially self-service off-licences and off-licences in supermarkets (see page 119), and that alcohol should not be allowed to become cheaper in real terms. Their recommendations on education were sensitive and sensible, advocating that the aim of education should be to encourage 'moderate drinking only in the appropriate circumstances and the acceptance of abstinence'. They also recommended that the attractive image of alcohol should be countered to provide a more balanced image reflecting its power to impair and harm, as well as its beneficial properties. Equal emphasis in the report was given to secondary prevention, the need to provide services which would try to offer those who were prepared to recognize that they were developing a serious drinking problem help in controlling their drinking before they progressed too far.

The government White Paper *Prevention and Health* endorsed

these recommendations, with the exception of that which called for the maintenance of the real price of alcohol by the use of taxation. In spite of the fact that the 'price' of a bottle of whisky fell from 569 minutes of manual work in 1950 to 209 minutes in 1976 while the 'price' of a loaf rose from 9 to 11 minutes, the government committed itself to no more than a promise that it would 'encourage public debate' and would keep the possibility under 'careful consideration'. The White Paper promised more support for health education, which spent less than £½ million in 1976 compared to the £36 million spent by the industry on television and in the press, and for research, for example on the identification of drinkers who might be more at risk. Alcohol presents a major challenge to prevention which is being taken up not only by public authorities, but by many other groups such as the National Council on Alcoholism and its local branches, the Medical Council on Alcoholism, the Alcohol Education Centre, the Teachers Advisory Centre on Drug and Alcohol Education, employers and trade unions, Alcoholics Anonymous, Al-Anon, the Christian Economic and Social Research Foundation, the United Kingdom Temperance Alliance Ltd., and the drinks industry itself. The industry's response to the problem is varied. Some firms are cautious, others like Whitbreads, Teacher's Whisky, the Scotch Whisky Association, and the Brewers Society have taken a keen interest in prevention and research, the latter tend to support the Medical Council on Alcoholism, but the general trend is towards involvement in prevention both in Britain and America (see page 136). Alcohol is a valuable, socially acceptable drug, but its side-effects are serious and have to be controlled. Because treatment of serious chronic problems rarely leads to a cure, the emphasis must be on prevention by the control of excess and encouragement of moderation. The Advisory Committee on Alcoholism emphasized the importance of this approach but they also recommended, in their second report on the pattern and range of services for problem drinkers which was published in 1978, that it was necessary to expand services so that help could be offered to more people at an earlier stage in their problem when the probability of success was higher.

Health and safety at work

In this field of preventive medicine legislation plays, and has played, a prominent part. In the nineteenth century the focus was on the working conditions of children and women. Peel's Act of 1802 covered only the health of apprentices: the Factory Act of 1819 extended the protection of the law to other young workers and proscribed work for children under nine years of age; the 1833 Factory Act introduced government inspection to enforce health and safety legislation; the 1844 Factory Act required, for the first time, that machinery should be enclosed, and subsequent acts extended the power of the law to protect child and women workers. As these abuses were mitigated, attention turned to the problems of working men and a whole series of Acts were passed covering four main areas of work: Factory Acts; Mines and Quarries Acts; Agricultural Acts; and the Offices, Shops, and Railway Premises Act. There were also Acts which dealt with dangerous substances, for example the Explosives Act of 1875, Hydrogen Cyanide (Fumigation) Act of 1937, and the Radioactive Substance Act of 1960; and Acts which are drafted to protect the public from environmental pollution, for example the Alkali etc., Works Regulation Act of 1906. A tremendous amount of legislation was placed on the Statute Books which was described in caustic prose by Sidney Webb in his Introduction to *A History of Factory Legislation in 1910*:

This century of experiment in factory legislation affords a typical example of English practical empiricism. We began with no abstract theory of social justice or the rights of man. We seem always to have been incapable even of taking a general view of the subject we were legislating upon. Each successive statute aimed at remedying a single ascertained evil. It was in vain that objectors urged that other evils, no more defensible, existed in other trades or amongst other classes, or with persons of ages other than those to which the particular Bill applied. Neither logic nor consistency, neither the over-nice consideration of even-handed justice nor the quixotic appeal of a general humanitarianism, was permitted to stand in the way of a practical remedy for a proved wrong.

The result of all this legislative activity was not only to build up an extremely complicated set of laws, but the establishment of a number of enforcing agencies; such as the Factory Inspectorate, the Mines and Quarries Inspectorate, the Explosives Inspectorate, the Nuclear Installations Inspectorate, the Alkali and Clean Air Inspectorate, all controlled by different parts of central government, together with the local authorities which had also been given certain responsibilities. To review this web of legislation and maze of bureaucracy the Robens Committee was appointed in 1970 and its report 'Safety and Health at Work', presented to Parliament in 1972, led to the Health and Safety at Work Act of 1974.

This consolidated many of the preceding Acts and laid down the general principles on which laws, regulations, and practices were to be based. It stated that 'it shall be the duty of every employer to ensure, so far as is reasonably practicable, the health, safety, and welfare at work of all his employees . . . the provision and maintenance of plant and systems of work that are safe and without risks to health . . . the provision of such information, instruction, training and supervision as is necessary to ensure the health and safety at work of his employees'. Section seven of the Act was equally forthright on the 'duty of every employee while at work to take reasonable care for the health and safety of himself and of other persons who may be affected by his acts or omissions' and to co-operate with his employer's health and safety policies.

Broad principles were set out clearly and boldly, and Sidney Webb would have been satisfied. To implement them the Act instituted a central, co-ordinating Health and Safety Commission consisting of members appointed from the C.B.I., the T.U.C., and local authorities. The Commission is served by the full-time staff of the Health and Safety Executive which consists of various policy divisions and all the inspectorates, which are either integral parts of the Executive or are attached by agreement with the relevant government departments. The Executive incorporates the Employment Medical Advisory Service which employs more than two hundred doctors and nurses.

The manner in which the employer shall implement the Act was also clearly stated in Regulations laid before the House of Commons in 1978, and a Code of Practice which amplified these Regulations. The employer has to nominate safety officers to be responsible for the health and safety of employees if he is unable to be responsible for all employees himself. These safety officers are usually the heads of the firm's departments and they may be assisted and advised by a full-time safety officer if the employer feels that he requires such specialist advice. To consider the employee's interests trade unions may nominate safety representatives, who may

- investigate potential hazards
- investigate complaints by any employee they represent relating to that employee's health and safety
- conduct regular inspections and carry out a special inspection where an accident or notifiable industrial disease has occurred
- represent the interests of those employees they represent to the safety officers and the management through a safety committee.

A safety committee, consisting of safety officers, safety represent-atives, managers, works doctors, and any other appropriate persons, may be set up if two or more safety representatives request it. The function of a safety committee is to consider the health and safety of the working environment by considering the statistics relating to accidents and disease, the reports of safety representatives, Health and Safety Executive inspectors, and any other pertinent source of information. The employer has to develop a safety policy for the work place.

The Act has many good aspects: the consolidating sections of the Act bring together the various inspectorates previously responsible for dangerous substances and environmental pollution and should lead to more effective control of physical and chemical hazards to health at work and in the community. More that eight million workers are now covered by health and safety legislation who had no cover under previous legislation. However, these sections of the Act which were intended to promote health and safety have given rise to difficulties. Not only have there been problems in the interpretation of the phrase 'so far as is reasonably practicable', but the style of the Act has given rise to more fundamental problems. The Act which was intended to be comprehensive has, in some organizations, appeared to have had little immediate beneficial effect on the employee's health and safety. The Act places the responsibility on the employer and on the head of each department but in complex organizations, such as hospitals, it has sometimes proved difficult to establish who the head actually is. If a hospital porter slips on a newly washed ward floor and fractures his wrist, who is responsible? The head porter who failed to train him adequately on the dangers of wet floors? Himself for not following his training? The housekeeper responsible for the work of domestics in her department? The sister in charge of the ward nursing staff? Or the consultant responsible for patient care? In universities the same problem has arisen when a professor is titular head of a department but the chief technician is in charge of work in the laboratories. Difficulties in the implementation of Acts are not uncommon if they were badly drafted, but the difficulties relating to the Health and Safety at Work Act of 1974 are, perhaps, not so much due to faults in the wording but in its very style. Whereas previous Acts dealt with the prevention of specific problems in identifiable places of types of work, or covered definable substances and omissions, this Act also deals with the promotion of health, which is virtually undefinable. The Health and Safety at Work Act, especially the statement of general principles, satisfies Sidney Webb's Platonic criteria but the benefits of dealing with each 'single ascertained evil' as it is detected, in an empirical fashion, should not be underestimated. Practical remedies for proven wrongs make for piecemeal and untidy legislation, but that may be a better approach to social policy than a more Utopian style of state intervention.

It will take, however, many years before the effectiveness of the Act can be judged. It did not come into force until January 1975, and it will take some time before all aspects of this complex law will be fully understood, as some sections have already required testing in the Courts to determine how they should be interpreted in practice. If the success or failure of such a broadly based Act and especially of the 1975 Safety Representative Regulations can be said to hinge on one factor, that factor is probably the attitudes of both employees and managers towards the opportunities for participation in health and safety policy-making which the Act offers. The Act has to be considered in the context of such legislation as the Trade Union and Labour Relations Act 1974, and the Employment Protection Act 1975, and the many other steps taken in the early 1970s towards increased worker participation. In the past the implicit principle underlying health and safety legislation was that the responsibility was primarily and correctly the employer's, but workers can often see problems and practices which should be corrected to prevent accidents and disease before managers and employers. To prevent accidents (see page 99) and illnesses in the work environments of the future, which may be free of the obvious dangers and hazards common in times past but which may harbour just as great, though less obvious, dangers, will require the full participation of those most intimately involved with the processes of work—the employees—and those who can prevent dangers during the planning stage—the managers.

Changes in attitude alone will not be sufficient. There is a need to increase the number of specially trained occupational health doctors and nurses and to give them the necessary facilities and co-operation to use their skills to prevent illness at work. The discussion paper *Occupational Health Services—The Way Ahead* published by the Health and Safety Commission in 1977, outlines the shortage of and reason for such services. The Act will entail expense. Local Authorities estimated in 1976 that the costs, principally the cost of releasing staff to be trained to fulfil their duties as safety representatives, would be between forty and eighty million pounds. In spite of the reservations expressed in this chapter it seems preferable that the Health and Safety at Work Act is the opening of a new and important chapter in preventive medicine.

9 The future of preventive medicine

There are hopeful portents for the future—in particular, the decline of cigarette smoking (see page 160) although it is a growing problem in underdeveloped countries. That the tobacco industry is aware of this trend is evident not only by its nervous mood—in 1978, full page advertisements were taken in *The Times* and *Financial Times* attacking those who sought greater controls on tobacco advertising— but also in the diversification of the tobacco companies. In 1978, British American Tobacco bought a paper-making company for 153 million dollars, although more than half of its profits in 1977 still came from tobacco. More significantly, in the same year (1977) Imperial Tobacco announced for the first time that more than half its profit derived from activities other than those concerned with tobacco: 53.9 per cent in comparison with only 46.3 per cent in 1976 and 43 per cent in 1975. The cigarette producers are aware of the turning tide. The control of cigarette smoking offers an example of another aspect of prevention which will become increasingly important—the influence of Britain's membership of the E.E.C..

In January 1978, Britain had to comply with the E.E.C. regulations on tobacco tax. The effect of such a change, if it had been implemented, would have been to reduce the difference in cost between small, tipped cigarettes and large, untipped cigarettes from 20 pence to 8 pence. However, Imperial Tobacco, to its credit, decided to adjust its prices to maintain this differential, thus co-operating with the government's aim of encouraging people to smoke low-tar cigarettes. Both these moves are significant; the tobacco company's action because it indicates its willingness to comply with government intentions, although not legally obliged to do so; the E.E.C.'s decision because it shows that Britain's approach to prevention will be modified by its Common Market membership. In some spheres E.E.C. influence will be beneficial— for example in its approach to consumer safety (see page 134); in other spheres, as in cigarette smoking, it will not be so. Whether or not the influence of the Community is regarded as helpful, it seems certain that the scope for unilateral legislative action is diminishing.

Other problems seem bound to arise, particularly those caused by man's wish to control the environment. Since man first tried to free himself from the exigencies of nature by wearing clothes, building dwellings, making fire, and domesticating animals, nature has waned as a threat to health but man's own activities have posed an ever-increasing threat. Each new ecosystem spawns new problems. Urbanization, irrigation, and industrialization, for example, have all conferred ecological advantages and disadvantages, and the rapid growth of chemical technology, which underpins almost every advance, is creating new problems.

The American Environment Protection Agency has estimated that there are 50,000 chemicals in everyday use, together with 1,500 pesticide chemicals, 4,000 active drug ingredients, and 7,500 chemicals added to foodstuffs, with new chemicals being developed every day. The possibility that a chemical might cause cancer can be tested either by using mice—the procedure taking months and costing 150,000 dollars, or by the Ames test, which uses recombinant DNA, takes two days, and costs 250 dollars. However, the Ames test is itself condemned as a danger by The Friends Of The Earth, who welcome the moves to test existing and new chemicals for their cancer risk, but fear that the recombinant DNA could lead to the evolution of new and lethal forms of bacteria. This is the crux of the dilemma. The greatest hazards may well come not from the use of technology for personal gain as a means of achieving power, but from attempts to feed more of the world's population, cure more diseases, and prevent cancer. In future, preventive medicine will not only have to develop its personal preventive programmes, dealing with smoking, obesity, alcohol abuse, and similar problems but it will have also to expand its ecological approach to protect man from actions of other men; actions which are inspired by their good intentions and their wish to improve the human condition.

The attempts to harness nuclear power offer a paradigm of the ecological dilemma. The malevolent use of nuclear power is an obvious threat but its benevolent use also entails risk. Britain is currently faced with the problem of the disposal of nuclear waste which will emit alpha particles for 100,000 years. The dangers inherent in this process may be prevented if the problem of nuclear fission is solved, but that may bring its own noxious side-effects.

Successive governments have recognized the importance of these developments and the Royal Commission on Environmental Pollution, which was instituted in 1970, produced six reports between 1971 and 1976 covering topics such as air pollution, the disposal of toxic industrial wastes, pollution in estuaries and coastal waters, radioactivity, and the problems of pollution control—for there are considerable problems. A shortage of skilled personnel and limited financial resources prevent effective environmental monitoring. In 1978, the Association of Public Analysts spelled out a warning in a report describing their poorly staffed and ill-equipped laboratories, highlighting the problems which have to be overcome.

The Department of the Environment's Central Unit on Environmental Pollution has produced an excellent series of 'Pollution Papers', but unless there is an adequately funded system of monitoring at local level to implement central policies, pollution may go undetected until it reaches dangerous levels. Adequate training and retraining of environmental health officers and ecologists, and the provision of suitable laboratory services are essential if diseases caused by chemical and radioactive substances are to be prevented.

Noise is another environmental problem which is increasing in severity. Although noise cannot be said to cause fatal diseases in the way in which asbestos and radioactive material can, it can cause deafness and aggravate mental disorder, and it greatly affects the quality of life. The Noise Advisory Council, which, like the Clean Air Council, is closely linked with the Department of the Environment, has issued reports on a variety of topics, particularly those concerned with aircraft noise. What has become apparent, again particularly in relation to aircraft noise and the siting of airfields, has been the rise of the consumer movement in public health, although it is not so well organized in Britain as in America. In 1978, the Centre for Auto Safety (C.A.S.), established by Ralph Nader in 1970, brought an £8.3 million suit against British Leyland for alleged safety defects in its cars. C.A.S. frequently petitioned the American government which then introduced regulations on, for example, energy absorbing steering-columns, the flammability of cars' interiors, and other safety features. As a result of the recommendations of the Pearson Report (see page 93), the Law Commission, an E.E.C. draft directive, and the Strasbourg Convention in 1978 it seems probable that manufacturers will be held liable for death or injury caused by defective products, without the need to prove negligence as is the case at present. If such an Act is passed, the power of the consumer movement will be greatly increased, as will its ability to influence the design and standards of products to ensure a greater degree of safety.

The quality of life has become an important political issue. In Europe, ecology parties are fighting for, and winning, votes and their concern, like that of ecologists in Britain and America, is with both the physical and social environment. Opposition to an energy strategy based on nuclear fuels is founded not only on the possibility of radioactive pollution, but also on the fact that such a system, on a grid of a few large power stations, increases the potency of central government and diminishes the significance of small groups and individuals. The ecological movement is con-cerned not only with the prevention of pollution but also with a political problem—the centralization of power. The ecological debate in Britain has been conducted more peacefully than in other countries. The calm reception of Mr. Justice Parker's 'Windscale Inquiry' into the reprocessing of nuclear waste, published by the Stationery Office in 1978, and the moderate approach of Friends of the Earth and the Conservation Society, contrasts with the strife in France and Germany over nuclear power stations, but it is probable that the reaction to such policies and plans will become stronger and more violent in all developed countries.

Diseases cannot be considered in isolation: their prevention has to be attempted in the context of the society in which they occur and in accordance with the wishes of individuals. Man does not only wish for freedom from pain, disability and premature death. He also wishes for freedom from anxiety and from interference by the State. Yet anxiety is inevitable if individuals are to be warned about possible hazards, and State interference inevitable in the prevention of disease. A balance of these freedoms has to be achieved, and this places prevention in politics just as much as in medicine.

Further reading

Chapter 1

The *Pelican Economic History of Britain* provides an excellent introduction to social history: Volume 1 is *The Medieval Economy and Society* by M. M. Postan (Penguin, 1975), Volume 2, *Reformation to Industrial Revolution* by C. Hill (Penguin, 1969), and Volume 3, *Industry and Empire* by E. J. Hobsbawm (Penguin, 1969). Professor Postan's book is particularly relevant to the social history of preventive medicine, describing in detail the factors leading to the change in the British diet and the fluctuations in population.

In *Plagues and People* (Blackwell, 1977) W. H. McNeil examines the epidemics of disease which have affected man, producing evidence to show how frequently man has created the conditions which caused the epidemics; Chapter IV, 'The Impact of the Mongol Empire on Shifting Disease Balances 1200–1500' discusses plague and leprosy in detail. *Food in History* (Eyre Methuen, 1973) by R. Tannahill describes the factors which have led to the improvement in man's nutritional status—Part IV, 'Europe A.D. 1000–1500', is of particular interest. In *The Black Death* (Collins, 1969) P. Ziegler traces the rising decline of plague in Europe. The fear generated by the plague is captured in *The Black Death—A Chronicle of the Plague Compiled from Contemporary Sources* (Allen and Unwin, 1926) by J. Nohl and in *A Journal of the Plague Year* (Penguin, 1966), which Daniel Defoe published in 1722. *Smallpox* (J. and A. Churchill, 1962) by C. W. Dixon includes an excellent history of vaccination.

The White Plague: Tuberculosis, Man, and Society (Little, Brown, 1953) by R. and J. Dubos describes the interesting social history of this disease. R. J. Morris gives an account of the first British cholera epidemic in *Cholera 1832* (Croom Helm, 1977) and N. Longmate gives an account of all the British epidemics in *King Cholera: The biography of a disease* (Hamish Hamilton, 1966). Both books describe the public and political reaction to cholera. T. McKeown's theories on the decline in mortality during the nineteenth and twentieth centuries are summarized in Chapters 1 and 8 of *An Introduction to Social Medicine* (Blackwell, 1974), which he wrote with C. R. Lowe. *Man, Environment and Disease in Britain: A Medical Geography through the ages* (Penguin, 1976) is a useful book, surveying much of the material concerned in this chapter, written by G. M. Howe.

Chapter 2

In *Effectiveness and Efficiency, Random Reflections on Health Services* (Nuffield Provincial Hospitals Trust, 1972) A. L. Cochrane rigorously reviews the evidence on the effectiveness of clinical medicine, and his conclusions suggest that it has been less effective than was generally assumed before the introduction of statistical evaluation. In *Statistical Methods in Medical Research* (Blackwell, 1971) P. Armitage sets out the statistical techniques in common use. Their practical application is described by D. J. P. Barker and G. Rose in *Epidemiology in Medical Practice* (Churchill Livingstone, 1976). The possible preventive measures for all the common infectious diseases in the world are clearly reviewed in the American Public Health Association's book *Control of Communicable Diseases in Man* (12th Edition 1975) edited by A. S. Benenson, which reveals the wide variation in the modes of human infection.

Chapter 3

In *The Population Bomb* (Pan, 1972) P. R. Ehrlich examines the implications of world population growth. Gunner Myrdhal's elegant analysis of poverty in *Asian Drama* (Allen Lane, 1968) is still pertinent and is complemented by a more recent study of the poverty of and within underdeveloped countries—*How the Other Half Dies* (Penguin, 1976) by S. George. Many of the medical text-books published for those working in developing countries illuminate the principles of prevention by education and by the early detection of the common treatable diseases. Notable among these texts are *Primary Child Care: A Manual for Health Workers* by M. and F. King and S. Martodipoero (O.U.P., 1978) and *Medical Care in Developing Countries: A Primer on the Medicine of Poverty and a Symposium from Makerere* edited by M. H. King (O.U.P., 1967).

Chapter 4

Prevention and Health: Everybody's Business, and the discussion paper *Reducing the Risk*, both produced by the Department of Health; the House of Commons Expenditure Committee's Report on *Preventive Medicine* and the White Paper *Prevention and Health* all discuss prevention in childhood. The Court Report *Fit for the Future, the Report of the Committee on Child Health Services* (Cmnd. 6684, H.M.S.O., 1974) and the Warnock Report on *Special Educational Needs, the Report of the Committee of Enquiry into the Education of Handicapped Children and Young People* (Cmnd. 7212, H.M.S.O., 1978) contain much useful information about the changing pattern of childhood disease and disability. The prevention of accidents is discussed in a series of papers edited by R. H. Jackson and published as *Children, the Environment and Accidents* (Pitman Medical, 1977). The pattern of deprivation revealed by the National Child Development Study (see page 59) is succinctly summarized in *Born to Fail* (Arrow, 1973) by P. Wedge and H. Prosser.

Chapter 5

The Report of the British Cardiac Society and the Royal College of Physicians on *The Prevention of Coronary Heart Disease* (Royal College of Physicians, 1976) reviews all the evidence in this field. Sir Richard Doll's book *Prevention of Cancer: Pointers from Epidemology* (Nuffield Provincial Hospitals Trust), although published in 1967, is a classic work elegantly describing not only possibilities for the prevention of cancer but the epidemiological approach. The British Chest, Heart, and Stroke Association, Tavistock House, Tavistock Square, London WC1, publish material on chest disease and strokes.

Social Trends (H.M.S.O., annually) includes data on all causes of death, with a separate section on accidents at home and at work. The Department of Transport and RoSPA produce periodic reports on road accidents. E. Stengel summarizes current data and theories about *Suicide and Attempted Suicide* (Penguin, 1964) lucidly.

The report of the social survey conducted by Amelia Harris of the Office of Population Censuses and Surveys, *Handicapped and Impaired in Great Britain* (H.M.S.O. 1971) discusses the common causes of disability and handicap and the problems of disabled people. Provocative, albeit minority, views on the nature of mental illness have been proposed by R. D. Laing in *The Divided Self* (Penguin, 1960) and T. Szasz in *The Myth of Mental Illness* (Paladin, 1962). A more conventional approach, and a refutation of their hypotheses, is presented by J. K. Wing in *Reasoning About Madness* (O.U.P., 1978). Exciting possibilities for the prevention of depression are suggested in *Social Origins of Depression, a Study of Psychiatric Disorder in Women* by G. W. Brown and T. Harris (Tavistock, 1978). *The Diseases of Occupations* (English University Press, 1975) by Donald Hunter comprehensively covers the diseases associated with working conditions. A survey by J. Martin and M. Morgan, from the Office of Population Censuses and Surveys, analyses the reasons for *Prolonged Sickness Absence and the Return to Work* (H.M.S.O. 1975). Other data on sickness absence from work are included in the Report of the Chief Medical Officer *On the State of the Public Health* (H.M.S.O. annually). *Alcoholism* (Penguin, 1965) by N. Kessel and H. Walton is useful reading. *Adolescents and Alcohol* (Edsall and Co., 1978) by A. Hawker describes this particular phenomenon with insight based on original research, and there are many interesting essays in *Notes on Alcohol and Alcoholism* (Medical Council on Alcoholism, 1975) which cover the most important aspects of the problems caused by alcohol. *The Non-Medical Use of Drugs* (Penguin, 1971), the interim report of the Canadian Government's Commission of Inquiry, is a comprehensive introduction to this subject. In *The Drugtakers* (Paladin, 1971), J. Young considers the social meaning of drug use in more detail.

A Happier Old Age (H.M.S.O., 1978), the Department of Health's discussion document and *The Elderly At Home* (H.M.S.O., 1977) review the problems of old people and their supporters.

Fluoride, Teeth and Health (Pitman Medical, 1976) is the report of the Royal College of Physicians on fluoridation. *Eating for Health* (Stationery Office, 1978) was published as a discussion document about the national diet.

Chapter 6

Acts of Parliament are bound in the volumes of *Public and General Acts and Measures* with the *Index to the Statutes* bound separately. They are kept by the larger public libraries as are the Regulations made under Act of Parliament which are bound in *Statutory Instruments*, with its separate *Index to Government Orders*. The major points of law affecting safety on the road are summarized at the end of the *Highway Code* (pages 61–8). *Clays Handbook of Environmental Health* (H. K. Lewis, 1977) is the standard text in this field, covering public health law, housing and urban development, pollution, and food hygiene.

On the reference shelves of public libraries at shelf marks 613 and 614 are gathered the more important public health reports, Statutory Instruments and Acts.

The British Standards Institution's publications describe their system of testing, control, and labelling and *Which*, the journal of the Consumers' Association, often has articles in which the safety of consumer goods is discussed.

The publications of the Ministry of Agriculture, Fisheries, and Food and the Department of Agriculture and Fisheries for Scotland —listed in *H.M.S.O. Sectional List 1*—describe the legislation controlling food standards and additives.

The Department of Education and Science publication *Health Education in Schools* (H.M.S.O., 1977) is the best introduction to this subject. *The Foundations and Principles of Health Education* (J. Wiley, 1978) by N. Galli examines the theoretical framework of health education.

Decoding Advertisements—Ideology and Meaning in Advertising (Marion Boyars, 1978) is a sound analysis of the techniques of advertising by J. Williamson; *Ethics, Economics, Effects: The Three Faces of Advertising* (The Advertising Association, 1975) is an interesting collection of essays, edited by Michael Barnes, written both by supporters of advertising and those who are critical of its effects.

The principles and practice of screening are discussed in *Prevention and Health: Everybody's Business* (op. cit.). Breast screening is considered in more detail in the White Paper *Prevention and Health* (op. cit.) and screening in pregnancy and childhood in *Reducing the Risk: Safer Pregnancy and Childbirth* (op. cit.).

Chapter 7

The linguistic theories of Benjamin Lee Whorfe are presented in a collection of his major essays *Language, Thought and Reality* (M.I.T.

Press, 1956) edited by J. B. Carroll. *The Uses of Literacy* (Allen Lane, 1957) by Richard Hoggart is a brillant analysis of the cultural and linguistic diversity in Britain. The manner in which individuals make decisions about risks is analysed by J. Cohen in *Psychological Probability and the Art of Doubt* (Allen and Unwin, 1972). The defences against anxiety which influence these decisions are described by E. Jaques in 'Social Systems as a Defence against Persecutions and Depressive Anxiety', an essay in *New Directions in Psychoanalysis* (Tavistock, 1955) and they are illuminated by K. Thomas's historical study of anxiety management, *Religion and the Decline of Magic* (Penguin, 1972). *Aggression on the Roads* (Tavistock Publications, 1968) by M. H. Perry considers the anxiety and aggression of road users and their influence on accident proneness.

The financial obstacles to prevention are described in *Prevention and Health: Everybody's Business*. Cost-benefit analysis is also the subject of part of Lord Ashby's excellent book *Reconciling Man and the Environment* (OUP,1978) and is discussed in *Cost-Benefit Analysis* (Penguin, 1972) edited by R. Layard. *The Value of Life* (Martin Robertson, 1976) by M. W. Jones-Lee is a econometric approach towards the assessment of the costs of premature death. *The Money Value of a Man* (Arno Press, 1977) by L. I. Dublin and A. J. Lotka summarizes the actuarial approach, both the authors being statisticians with the Metropolitan Life Insurance Company.

The relationship of the State and the individual as expressed by the role of law has always been a central theme of political philosophy. One of the most important influences on British jurisprudence is still *On Liberty*, written in 1859 by J. S. Mill, which was itself influenced by *The Limits of State Action* by a German, Wilhelm von Humboldt, which was written in 1891–2. In the 1960s interest in the role of law was reactivated by the conflicting opinions of H. L. A. Hart, as expressed in *Law, Liberty, and Morality* (O.U.P., 1963) and Lord Devlin in *The Enforcement of Morals* (O.U.P., 1965). An excellent summary of this debate is provided by the series of essays published as *The Philosophy of Law* (O.U.P., 1977) edited by R. M. Dworkin whose own contribution synthesises the two opposing schools of thought. *The State, Society and Self-Destruction* (Allen and Unwin, 1975), a series of essays edited by E. Vallance, examines the particular aspect of the legislative control of drugs. A broader philosophical view of life, death, and liberty is given by J. Glover in

Causing Death and Saving Lives (Penguin, 1977) and by Isaiah Berlin in his brilliant essay 'Two Concepts of Liberty' in *Four Essays on Liberty* (O.U.P., 1969).

Chapter 8

The White Paper *Prevention and Health* (H.M.S.O., 1977) covers the strategy for the prevention of diseases caused by cigarette smoking in considerable detail. The White Paper also discusses, although in less detail, the prevention of problems caused by alcohol abuse. (See also the references for Chapter 5.) The Department of Health's Advisory Committee on Alcoholism reports on *Prevention* (H.M.S.O., 1977) and on the *Pattern and range of services for problem drinkers* (H.M.S.O., 1978) are excellent summary papers. The Department of Employment and the Health and Safety Commission, catalogued separately in public libraries, publish material on the promotion of health and safety at work. *Occupational Health services: The Way Ahead* (H.M.S.O., 1977) is an important booklet on this topic. Others cover dangers at work and the prevention of industrial diseases and accidents.

Chapter 9

The principles of ecology are outlined in *What is Ecology?* (O.U.P., 1974) by D. F. Owen, who also illustrates the ecological approach in *Man's Environmental Predicament: An Introduction to Human Ecology in Africa* (O.U.P., 1978). Lord Ashby presents the manner in which society and politicians regard the risks of pollution in *Reconciling Man with the Environment* (O.U.P., 1978), a clear and comprehensive analysis. The problems of environmental pollution and its control is well reported by J. Bugler in *Polluting Britain* (Penguin, 1972).

Unsafe at Any Speed—The Designed-in Dangers of the American Automobile (Grossman, 1965) epitomizes the style of consumer pressure pioneered by the author, Ralph Nader. The consultative document *Consumer Safety* (Cmnd. 6398, H.M.S.O., 1976) provides an interesting insight into the British Government's consumers' rights initiatives, and the report of *Royal Commission on Civil Liability and Compensation for Personal Injury* (Cmnd. 7054, H.M.S.O., 1978) discusses the principles on which consumer's rights and manufacture liability should be based. The evidence gathered in this three-volume report makes particularly interesting reading. Also published in 1978 in Britain were *The Social Audit Pollution Handbook: How to Assess Environmental and Workplace Pollution* by M. Frankel, and *The Social Audit Consumer Handbook: A Guide to the Social Responsibilities of Business to the Consumer* by C. Medawar (both Macmillan), to help individuals determine their rights and question the social responsibilities of the companies they work for, whose products they buy and whose factories are near their homes. H. A. Waldron's *The Medical Role in Environmental Health* (O.U.P./N.P.H.T., 1978) clearly reviews the development of environmental health services, and presents a useful survey of their problems.

Sources of personal advice

General practitioners and health visitors are the principal advisers on prevention. They receive much of their material from health education officers who are employed by the area health authorities (in Scotland area health boards). Health education officers can be approached directly by members of the public but their service is often aimed more at those who might be advising others, for example, school teachers or youth workers, than at individual members of the public. The Health Education Council, 78 New Oxford Street, London WC1A, or the Scottish Health Education Unit, 21 Lansdowne Crescent, Edinburgh EH12 5EN, publish a number of leaflets and booklets and both have a wide range of films which can be borrowed.

Environmental health officers can advise on home safety and environmental problems, such as noise and smoke. Road safety training officers are employed by county councils, and fire department staff can also be approached directly for advice. RoSPA, 4 Priory Queensway, Birmingham B4 6BS, is interested in the prevention of all types of accidents. If it is not clear whom to consult concerning health and safety at work, the personnel department should be approached.

Government papers

Each year the Chief Medical Officer of the Department of Health publishes an annual report entitled *On The State of the Public Health* and the Secretary of State for Health and Social Services presents his *Annual Report* to Parliament. The emphasis of the former is on health problems while that of the latter is on health service problems, but the two are complementary. Health and social services statistics are published in separate volumes. A full list of the principal sources of official information is *Government Statistics—a brief guide to sources*, published annually by the Government Statistical Service. The publications of government departments and the larger agencies, such as the Health and Safety Executive, are collected in a series of Sectional Lists. *Social Trends,* which is another H.M.S.O. annual collates many of the important statistics from all government departments providing a useful background to the statistics relating particularly to illness.

The *Civil Service Yearbook* (H.M.S.O. annually) is a useful guide to the structure of central government and the functions of the various departments and their sections.

In 1976 the Health Departments of Great Britain and Northern Ireland published *Prevention and Health: Everybody's Business* which reviewed the major aspects of prevention in Britain. It was planned that a series of discussion papers were to follow this, of which the first two, *Reducing the Risk: Safer Pregnancy and Childbirth* and *Occupational Health Services: The Way Ahead*, appeared in 1977 and *Eating for Health* in 1978. In the same year the Social Services and Employment Sub-Committee of the Expenditure Committee of the House of Commons published its report on *Preventive Medicine* together with the evidence it had received. This was followed by the White Paper *Prevention and Health* (Cmnd. 247) which was presented to Parliament by the Secretaries of State for Health and Social Services, Education and Science, Scotland, and Wales.

Take Care of Yourself, A Practical Do-It-Yourself Guide to Medical Care (Allen & Unwin, 1979) by Donald M. Vickery, James F. Fries, J. A. Muir Gray, Simon A. Smail gives advice on the steps which individuals can take to prevent illness, guidance on how to use the full range of health services appropriately, and suggests ways of treating common illnesses at home.

Index

Accidents, in childhood, 57; to disadvantaged children, 60; farm, 155; home, 82–4, 121; loss of life from, 63; road traffic, 77–82; work, 100, 103, 106

Acts of Parliament, Agricultural (Acts), 167; Alkali, etc. Works Regulation, 1906, 167; Baths and Wash-houses, 1846, 120; Civil Registration, 1837, 1; Clean Air (Acts), 75; Consumer Protection, 1961, 121; Control of Pollution, 1974, 75; Customs and Excise, 1952, 120–1; Diseases of Animals (Acts), 121; Divorce Reform, 1969, 61; Education, 1907, 20; Education (Provision of Meals), 1906, 20; Employment Protection, 1975, 170; Explosives, 1875, 167; Factory (Acts), 167; Fire Precautions, 1971, 121; Food and Drugs, 1955, 121, 150; Health and Safety at Work, 1974, 134; Home Safety, 1961, 133; Hydrogen Cyanide (Fumigation), 1937, 167; Industrial Injuries, 1946, 104; Infectious Diseases, 1889, 19; Infectious Disease (Prevention), 1890, 120; Local Government, 1885, 19; Maternity and Child Welfare, 1918, 20; Medicines, 1968, 49; Metropolis Water, 1852, 19; Midwives, 1902, 20; Mines and Quarries (Acts), 167; Misuse of Drugs, 1971, 119; National Assistance, 1948, 14, 21; National Health Re-organization, 1973, 133; Notification of Births, 1915, 20; Nuisance Removal and Disease Prevention (Acts), 9, 17, 19; Offices, Shops, and Railway Premises, 1963, 167; Public Health of 1848, 19, 22; of 1871, 19; of 1872, 22; of 1875, 19; of 1936, 120; Public Health (Prevention and Treatment of Disease), 1913, 120; Radioactive Substances, 1960, 167; River Pollution Prevention, 1876, 120; Road Traffic of 1967, 81; of 1974, 134; Sanitary, 1866, 19; Trade Union and Labour Relations, 1975, 170; Vaccination (Acts), 10; Workmen's Compensation, 1897, 104

Adolescents, 61, 112

Advertising, 131–7; of cigarettes, 131–2, 135, 159, 162, 163; of alcohol, 131–2, 135–6

Advertising Standards Authority, 130, 135

Aetiology, 24

Age Concern, 122, 130

Air pollution, 74–5, 166

Al-Anon, 166

Alcohol, 111–12, 165–6; and foetal damage, 49; availability of, 119; and road traffic accidents, 80, 111, 136; taxation of, 116–8

Alcohol Education Centre, 166

Alcoholics Anonymous, 166

Alcoholism, 111, 112, 165–6; Advisory Committee on, 165–6; Medical Council on, 122, 166; National Council on, 166

Amniocentesis, 45

Amphetamines, 119

Anaesthesia, 3

Anderson, Sir Ferguson, 114

Anorexia Nervosa, 109

Anthropologist, 29

Antibiotics, 32–3, 57, 74

DATE DUE